MW00845292

The Invisible Light

The Invisible Light

100 YEARS OF
MEDICAL RADIOLOGY

EDITED BY

A.M.K. THOMAS

ASSISTED BY

I. ISHERWOOD & P.N.T. WELLS

**Blackwell
Science**

©1995 by
Blackwell Science Ltd
Editorial Offices:
Osney Mead, Oxford OX2 0EL
25 John Street, London WC1N 2BL
23 Ainslie Place, Edinburgh EH3 6AJ
238 Main Street, Cambridge
  Massachusetts 02142, USA
54 University Street, Carlton
  Victoria 3053, Australia

Other Editorial Offices:

Arnette Blackwell SA
1, rue de Lille, 75007 Paris, France

Blackwell Wissenschafts-Verlag GmbH
Kurfürstendamm 57, 10707 Berlin, Germany *and*
Feldgasse 13, A-1238 Wien, Austria

First published 1995

Set by Marksbury Typesetting Ltd, Midsomer Norton,
  Bath, UK
Printed at Alden Press Limited, Great Britain

DISTRIBUTORS

Marston Book Services Ltd
PO Box 87
Oxford OX2 0DT
(*Orders*: Tel: 01865 791155
         Fax: 01865 791927
         Telex: 837515)

North America
Blackwell Science, Inc.
238 Main Street
Cambridge, MA 02142
(*Orders*: Tel: 800 215-1000
         617 876-7000
         Fax: 617 492-5263)

Australia
Blackwell Science Pty Ltd
54 University Street
Carlton, Victoria 3053
(*Orders*: Tel: 03 347-0300
         Fax: 03 349-3016)

A catalogue record for this title
is available from the British Library
and the Library of Congress
ISBN 0 86542 627 9

Contents

v

Preface

The year 1995 commemorates two centenaries in connection with Willhelm Conrad Röntgen. The 8 November marks the centenary of his discovery of X-rays at Würzburg. The 27 March is the 150th anniversary of his birth at Lennep near Remscheid.

In June 1995 the various organizations concerned with Medical and Dental Radiology in the United Kingdom and Ireland collaborated in a major meeting held at the International Convention Centre and the National Indoor Arena in Birmingham, England. These organizations are the British Institute of Radiology, the College of Radiographers, the Faculty of Radiologists of the Royal College of Surgeons of Ireland, the Institute of Physical Science in Medicine, the Royal College of Nursing, the Royal College of Radiologists, the Section of Radiology of the Royal Society of Medicine and the Scottish Radiological Society.

The Röntgen Centenary Congress was initiated by the activities of the Radiology History and Heritage Charitable Trust, a multi-disciplinary group which encourages the study of the rich and complex story that is medical radiology. A group was assembled by the Röntgen Centenary Congress Committee to organise the Centenary Historical Exhibition entitled 'The Invisible Light, 100 years of Medical Radiology'. The majority of the authors of this book contributed to this Exhibition. The contributors are from diverse backgrounds and reflect the many different facets of radiology over the last 100 years. Each contributor has approached his or her task from their own particular viewpoint.

Medical radiology initially involved the use of X-rays for the diagnosis and treatment of disease. Becquerel then discovered radioactivity in 1897, and Marie Curie isolated radium in 1899. These newly discovered radioactive substances were almost immediately used in therapy and this remained the state of affairs for many years. Following the Second World War radionuclides were introduced into the medical diagnostic field and are now providing unique contributions to functional studies and molecular biology. Diagnostic ultrasound started in the 1950s and rapidly increased in use and diversity during the 1970s and 1980s. X-ray techniques, both diagnostic and interventional, have continued to develop with the introduction of image intensification in the 1960s and computed tomography scanning in the 1970s. More recently the phenomenon of nuclear magnetic resonance has been utilized in magnetic resonance imaging and magnetic resonance spectroscopy which have revolutionized our understanding of disease. Scientists in the United Kingdom have been in the forefront of all these radiological advances.

There can be few people now living in the United Kingdom who have not benefited either directly or indirectly from medical radiology at some point in their lives. The changes in technology in the last 100 years have been profound. Who knows what the next 100 years will bring?

For information about the Radiology History and Heritage Charitable Trust please contact: The Secretary, c/o The British Institute of Radiology, 36 Portland Place, London W1N 3DG

Adrian Thomas
Ian Isherwood
Peter Wells

Acknowledgements

The Rontgen Centenary Congress Committee would like to acknowledge the enormous support, both financial and technical, provided by Blackwell Science that make this publication possible. The editors would like particularly to thank Mr John Robson.

The Discovery of X-Rays and Radioactivity

Introduction

In the space of three years at the end of the last century, the major discoveries occurred of X-rays by Wilhelm Conrad Röntgen (November 1895), radioactivity by Henri Becquerel (March 1896) and radium by Marie & Pierre Curie (December 1898). This was to be the foundation of the science of medical radiology, both diagnostic and therapeutic, as well as of industrial radiography which today has applications in fields as varied as non-destructive testing of metal components, authentication of museum artefacts, airport security, and in the art world the study of paintings to detect changes made by the original artist and by restorers. These were three truly great discoveries which have in the 20th century had a vast impact on healthcare and on society in general.

X-rays

The first of these discoveries was made in Würzburg where Röntgen [1.1] had moved from Giessen in 1888. At the time he was investigating the phenomena caused by the passage of an electrical discharge from an induction coil through a partially-evacuated glass tube. The tube was completely covered with black paper and the whole room was in complete darkness, yet he observed that, elsewhere in the room, a paper screen covered with the fluorescent material barium platinocyanide became illuminated [1.2].

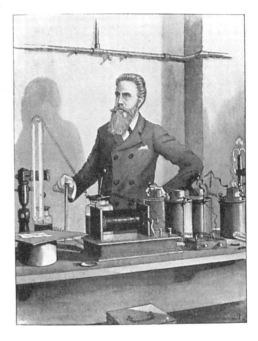

1.2 The world's first journalistic drawing of 'Röntgen at work'. It was published in the April 1896 issue of *The Windsor Magazine* in an article by the photographer Snowden Ward entitled 'Marvels of the new light'. However, there is a mistake: the tube shown is not the pear-shaped tube used in the discovery (courtesy: British Institute of Radiology).

It did not take him long to discover that not only black paper but other objects such as a wooden plank, a thick book and metal sheets, were also penetrated by these X-rays. In the words of his biographer Otto Glasser, he found that 'Strangest of all, while flesh was very transparent, bones were fairly opaque, and

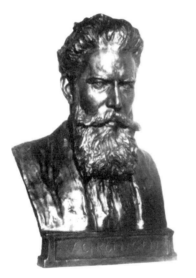

1.1 Bust of Röntgen (1845–1923) sculpted by Reinhold Felderhoff in 1896 (courtesy: Deutsches Röntgen Museum, Remscheid-Lennep).

interposing his hand between the source of the rays and his bit of luminescent cardboard, he saw the bones of his living hand projected in silhouette upon the screen. The great discovery was made'.

He notified several of his scientific colleagues, both in Germany and in other countries, of his results, sending them prints of his radiographs on 1 January 1896. In the United Kingdom this group of scientists included Sir Arthur Schuster in Manchester [1.3] and Lord Kelvin in Glasgow.

The response to what was often in 1896 referred to as 'the new light' was immediate and varied, from scientists recreating his experiments in private or university laboratories where the apparatus required was available, to the world's popular press making bizarre claims for X-rays. It was claimed, for example, that they were the philosopher's stone which could turn base metal to gold. Not only were the early newspaper reports often inaccurate as to the discovery and the possible uses, but they also initially misspelt Röntgen's name as Routgen

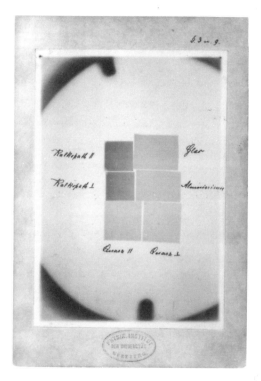

1.3 One of Röntgen's original 1895 radiographs showing absorption through equal thicknesses of different substances: glass, aluminium, calcite and quartz (courtesy: Wellcome Trustees).

and claimed that he worked in Vienna. Indeed, some of the 1896 textbooks on X-rays also made mistakes, for example printing the world's first cardiac image upside down and claiming that Röntgen was a Dutchman from Appeldoorn, where in fact he had only studied as a young man.

Public demonstrations and lectures became widespread [1.4, 1.5], although Röntgen himself only ever gave one presentation: on 23 January 1896, at the Physikalisch-medizinischen Gesellschaft in Würzburg. It was here that he radiographed the hand of von Kölliker [1.6], the anatomy professor in Würzburg, who proposed the term 'Röntgen rays' and called for three cheers for Röntgen. The audience cheered again and again.

Röntgen's first paper on X-rays was entitled *Ueber eine neue Art von Strahlen*, laid out in numbered paragraphs 1–17 and communicated on 28 December 1895. His second, on 9 March 1896 was a continuation of the first with additional numbered paragraphs 18–21. His third and final paper, for surprisingly he only ever published three on the subject of X-rays, was entitled 'Further observations on the properties of X-rays' was submitted on 10 March 1897 and published in *Annalen der Physik und Chemie* with an English translation in the February 1899 issue of *The Archives of the Roentgen Ray*.

X-ray therapy had its historical roots as early as 1896, when the Viennese dermatologist Leopold Freund treated a five-year old girl in November of that year. This was not for cancer but for epilation as she had a 36-cm hairy naevus on her back. Freund later recorded that 'In June 1896 I read in a Vienna newspaper the joke news that an American engineer who was intensively engaged in X-ray examinations lost his hair because of business'. However, the patient was not treated in a hospital, as none at the time would allow this, and the X-ray therapy was given at the Imperial and Royal Graphic School and Research Institute, directed by the photographer Eder who with Valenta produced in 1896 an album of excellent image quality radiographs: one copy of which was sent to Röntgen as a present and which is now in his old laboratory which houses a museum. This story, though, does not stop here. This five-year-old patient had a follow-up 70 years later where it was found that apart from back pain she was in good health. There had been no radiation-induced skin cancer.

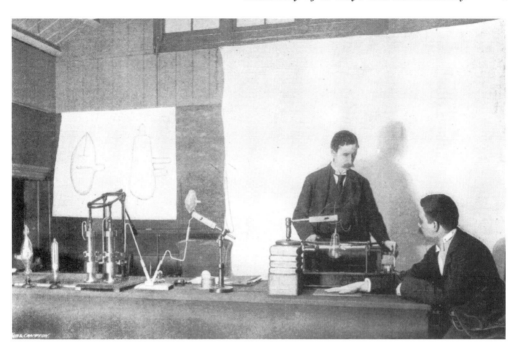

1.4 A.A. Campbell-Swinton, who is credited with making the first radiograph in the United Kingdom, 'surrounded by his apparatus as used in lecturing before the Royal Photographic Society'. This was taken in February 1896, the pear-shaped X-ray tube is clearly seen both in the wooden retort stand resting on a pile of books and on the illustration far left, and also appeared in *The Windsor Magazine* (courtesy: British Institute of Radiology).

In conclusion, Röntgen continued as Professor of Physics in Würzburg until 1900 when he left for the University of Munich. He was awarded the first Nobel Prize in Physics, in 1903, died in 1923 and is buried in the Röntgen family grave in Giessen.

Radioactivity

Following Röntgen's discovery, several scientists initially correlated fluorescence directly with the production of X-rays, and Henri Poincare suggested that it might be worthwhile investigating

1.5 Radiograph taken by Charles Thurston Holland in Liverpool on 22 October 1896: 3 minute exposure with a 6 in induction coil. He reported that someone had given him a small red brick to radiograph, stating that he had returned with it from Egypt and wondered if there was anything inside. A mummified bird was revealed. Egyptian mummies and small mammals such as frogs were often used as test objects, but in addition, there was a great interest in X-ray pictures of gems since the false could be quickly distinguished from the real.

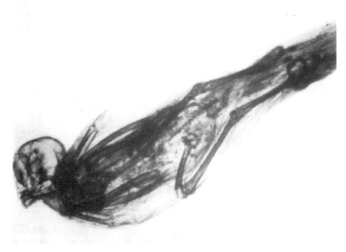

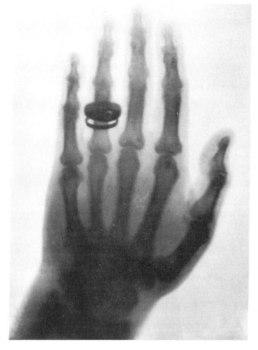

1.6 Hand of von Kolliker, taken by Röntgen on 23 January 1896, at the time of his one and only public lecture on X-rays (courtesy: Physical Institute, University of Würzburg).

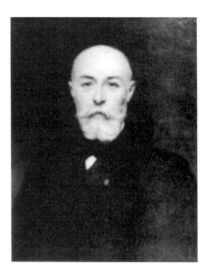

1.7 Henri Becquerel (1852–1908) (courtesy: Maria Sklodowska-Curie Museum, Warsaw).

whether or not rays similar to X-rays might be produced by ordinary fluorescent or phosphorescent substances. Henri Becquerel [1.7] followed this suggestion and placed fluorescent mineral crusts on photographic plates wrapped in light-tight black paper, exposed them to sunlight, and did observe an image on the plates.

On one occasion in February 1896 poor weather prevented exposure to sunlight and Becquerel put both the prepared plates and the minerals away in a drawer. On 1 March 1896 he removed them and, for some unknown reason, immediately developed the photographic plates before any exposure to sunlight.

To his surprise, he saw silhouetted images of the crust shapes on the developed plates. He concluded that neither sunlight, nor fluorescence nor phosphorescence was necessary to produce this effect. He also found that the radiation (initially called Becquerel rays) could penetrate thin strips of aluminium and copper as well as sheets of black paper.

He presented his discovery the following evening at the weekly Monday meeting of the French Academy of Sciences and publication of his paper followed within 10 days in *Comptes Rendus*, with the title 'On visible radiations emitted by phosphorescent bodies'. He later collaborated with the Curies and with them was jointly awarded the 1903 Nobel Prize for Physics. He died in 1908 at the age of 55 years.

Radium

The initial impetus for the discovery of radium was following the use of ionization methods to measure the intensity of X-rays. Marie Curie [1.8]

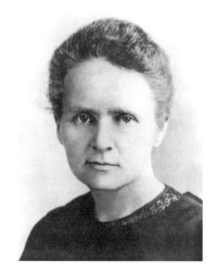

1.8 Maria Sklodowska-Curie (1867–1934) in 1923 (courtesy: Maria Sklodowska-Curie Museum, Warsaw).

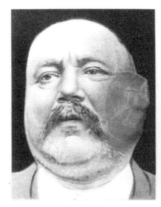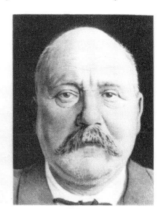

1.9 Patient with epithelioma of the parotid, 1905, Paris, before and after treatment. (Source: *Radiumtherapy* by Louis Wickham & Paul Degrais, Cassell:London, 1910).

realised that the radiations discovered by Becquerel could also be measured using ionization techniques which were a viable alternative to the photographic plate. She showed first that the radiation intensity was proportional to the amount of uranium but of the many substances studied, only thorium compounds were similar to uranium. It was then found that the uranium mineral pitchblende showed a higher radiation intensity than could be explained merely by the presence of uranium and thorium. In July 1898 the Curies discovered polonium (named for Marie Curie's country of birth:Poland) which was associated with the bismuth extract of pitchblende. Finally, in December the Curies discovered radium, which was associated with the barium extract of the ore. Nevertheless, it was an immense problem to refine it in any quantity and initially only one-tenth of a grain of radium could be extracted from two tons of pitchblende.

Tragically, Pierre Curie died in a road accident in 1906, at the early age of 47 years, but Marie Curie continued her scientific work which led not only to the rewards of two Nobel Prizes, one for physics and one for chemistry, but also the founding of two Radium Institutes: one in Paris (now the Institut Curie) and one in Poland (now the Maria Sklodowska-Curie Memorial Cancer Center and Institute of Oncology). Her gift of radium needles and tubes to the Polish Radium Institute are still in existence, although no longer used, and each is engraved with the initials RMS. In World War I she was the Director of the Red Cross Radiology Service, drove an ambulance in the front lines and was assisted by her daughter Irene, who with her husband Frederic Joliot in January

1934 discovered the phenomenon of artificial radioactivity. Sadly, Marie Curie died a few months later that year at the age of 67 years: her death was due to aplastic anaemia.

Radium sources were first used as surface plaques (termed moulds), not only for skin cancers but also for non-malignant conditions such as lupus. Some of the immediate effects on previously untreatable tumours, was dramatic [1.9] but it was soon realized that 'permanent' cures were not generally achievable. Up to 1904 radium was also studied as an alternative to X-rays for

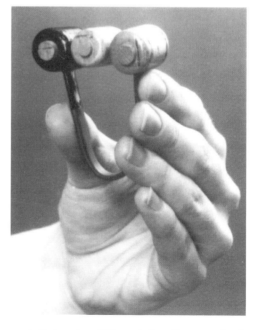

1.10 Paris system 1920s vaginal applicators made of cork cylinders into which were placed the radium sources. Two corks were joined together with a flexible spring.

diagnostic purposes and there is in existence a radiumgraph taken by Marie Curie of a purse and its contents. However, the lack of contrast due to the high gamma ray energy spectrum soon showed that radium as a diagnostic tool was unsuitable.

Following the use of surface moulds, the next development was intracavitary use of radium sources, mainly for cancer of the cervix, and by the 1920s three standard systems had been proposed with a large amount of success from Paris [1.10], Munich and Stockholm. By the early 1920s the interstitial use of radium needles was already established and by the end of the 1920s there was hardly a body site which had not had a radium or radon source treatment technique devised. The only notable exceptions in today's range of treatments are bile duct tumours which are only accessible using miniature iridium-192 high dose rate sources. It must also be remembered that the forerunner of the telecobalt-60 machines was the teleradium unit with sources which ranged from 1 g at the end of World War I to 10 g radium in the late 1950s. Radium was therefore a most important historical root for radiotherapy.

The Early Reception of Röntgen's Discovery in the United Kingdom

The Annus Mirabilis – 1896

'Progress is a thing of months and weeks, almost of days ... The suspense is becoming feverish.' Oliver Lodge, address to the Royal Institution, circa 1888.

News of the discovery of X-rays reached Britain in the first week of 1896 by two routes: Röntgen sent offprints of the paper describing his discovery to physicist friends Professors Arthur Schuster and Lord Kelvin at the New Year. Most people heard of it through the newspapers—foreign correspondents picked up the news from the Vienna paper *Neue Freie Presse* whose editor's son was a young physicist colleague of Franz Exner, another friend of Röntgen's who received an offprint. Robert Jones, the Liverpool surgeon, learnt about it from a neighbour who had relations in Vienna. He was probably the first doctor in Britain to know.

The short newspaper reports on 6, 7 and 8 January 1896 were factual and with little comment, but their significance was not lost on those who were familiar with recent experimental science. No previous scientific discovery had such a reception as greeted Röntgen's report.

The popular press, the world of science and the medical profession reacted with a mixture of amazement, incredulity and applause [2.1]. *The Times* ignored the subject. The *Lancet* was initially scathing, then factual and by the end of January enthusiastic. The photographic journals made much of the discovery, treating it as a branch of their own science. *Punch* of course poked fun, publishing a series of cartoons illustrating the feelings of the time. One entitled 'The New Photographic Discovery' [2.2] showed an accurate appreciation of the physical principles, in political guise. Another—'The March of Science' [2.3]—was more confused.

Four groups of people became involved in X-ray production during the first six months of 1896: academic physicists, scientific amateurs, men of commerce and doctors. Most appreciated the medical and surgical potential of the discovery and many became engaged in clinical radiography.

This was still an era in which gifted and wealthy amateurs, country parsons and school teachers were able to contribute to science. Amateur scientists, among them C.E.S. Phillips, J.W. Gifford and Lord Blythswood, tried their hands at the technique. Gifford and Blythswood were men of independent means whose science was a serious hobby. Both provided practical assistance to medical friends; Blythswood gave apparatus to the radiology department at Glasgow Royal Infirmary, Gifford X-rayed patients sent to him by the

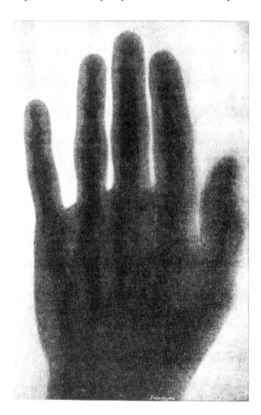

2.1 The first radiograph in the *British Medical Journal*, 25 January 1896. Taken by Alan Campbell Swinton.

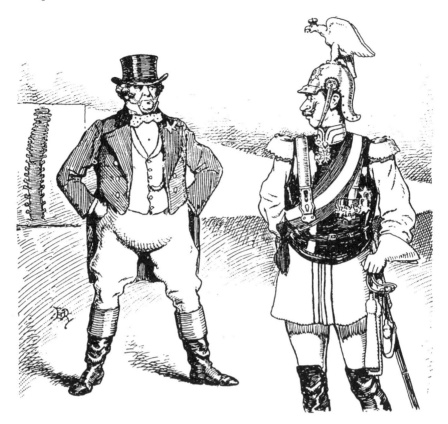

2.2 A cartoon from *Punch* 25 January 1896. The caption reads:

'THE NEW PHOTOGRAPHIC DISCOVERY
Thanks to the discovery of Professor Röntgen, the German Emperor will now be able to obtain an exact, photograph of a "back bone" of unsuspected size and strength.'

It was accompanied by the following poem:

THE NEW PHOTOGRAPHY

Professor Röntgen, of Würzburg, has discovered how to photograph through a person's body, giving a picture only of the bones.

O, Röntgen, then the news is true,
    And not a trick of idle rumour,
That bids us each beware of you,
    And of your grim and graveyard humour.

We do not want, like Dr. Swift,
    To take our flesh off and to pose in
Our bones, or show each little rift
    And joint for you to poke your nose in.

We only crave to contemplate
    Each other's usual full-dress photo;
Your worse than "altogether" state
    Of portraiture we bar *in toto*!

The fondest swain would scarcely prize
    A picture of his lady's framework;
To gaze on this with yearning eyes
    Would probably be voted tame work!

No, keep them for your epitaph,
    These tombstone-souvenirs unpleasant;
Or go away and photograph
    Mahatmas, spooks, and Mrs. B-s-nt!

doctors of Chard in Somerset where he lived. Reverend radiographers included Thomas Espin, vicar of Tow Law, whose experiments were published in the photographic journals, Frederick Walter, a minister in Norfolk, who took the first X-rays for his local hospital, and Brother Potamian O'Reilly DSc, maker of the first radiograph in Waterford, whose skill in physics and teaching soon gained him the position of head of engineering at Manhattan College, New York. H.S. Pyne, science master at King William's College, Isle of Man, used school equipment to photograph a frog before June 1896.

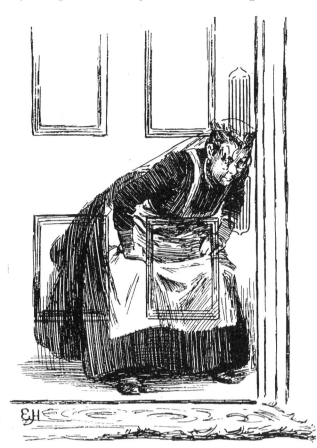

2.3 Another *Punch* cartoon from 7 March 1896 which had the following caption:

'THE MARCH OF SCIENCE
Interesting result attained, with aid of Röntgen rays, by a first-floor lodger when photographing his sitting-room door.'

As in Germany, there were physicists in Britain already working on the passage of electricity through a vacuum, including William Crookes, an independent scientist, Herbert Jackson of King's College, London and Arthur Schuster at Manchester. Others had or quickly assembled the necessary apparatus, such as Silvanus Thompson of Finsbury Technical College who was able to verify the existence of X-rays within days of the announcement.

Through public lectures, demonstrations and learned articles, academic scientists helped to spread knowledge of the discovery to doctors and a wider audience. Oliver Lodge lectured in Liverpool on 27 January, 3 and 24 February, S.P. Thompson at the Clinical Society of London in March, Schuster in Manchester the same month. The most influential publications were Arthur Stanton's translation of Röntgen's paper in *Nature* on 16 January, the radiograph of Swinton's hand printed in *Nature* on 23

January, and the series of articles by the medical student Sydney Rowland in the *British Medical Journal* throughout 1896 [2.4, 2.5].

Sidney Rowland had been appointed as the 'Special Commissioner to the *British Medical Journal* for the investigation of the application of the New Photography to Medicine and Surgery'. The quality of the radiographs is excellent and some were taken by Rowland himself at the Royal Free Hospital. Rowland also edited a new journal *The Archives of Clinical Skiagraphy* which first appeared in May 1896. This journal ultimately became the *British Journal of Radiology*.

Professors J.J. Thomson of Cambridge and Schuster of Manchester assisted medical practitioners to obtain X-rays, by making their laboratory equipment available. Physicist-doctor associations sprang up round British universities: Kelvin and John Macintyre in Glasgow, Oliver Lodge, Robert Jones and

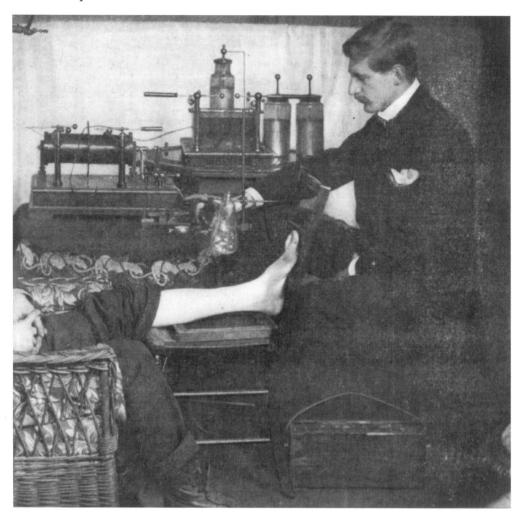

2.4 Photograph of patient being skiagraphed together with the apparatus necessary: radiography by Sidney Rowland (*British Medical Journal*, 29 February 1896)

Thurstan Holland in Liverpool, with less well-known links in Birmingham, Sheffield, New-castle, Manchester and London. Jones, Holland and Lodge met on 7 February to attempt a radiograph of a bullet in a boy's wrist. After failures, a two hour exposure secured a useful image which enabled the bullet to be removed.

Such personal association between scientists and doctors was short-lived, but the link between science and medicine was to be vital to the development of medical radiology in Britain. It was formally expressed in the first radiological association, the Röntgen Society, founded in 1897, where they, the engineers and the manufacturers met on equal terms. Silvanus

Thompson was the first President of the Röntgen Society which ultimately became the British Institute of Radiology and gave his Presidential address at its second meeting in St Martin's Town Hall on November 5th 1897.

Prominent among the men of commerce was A.A. Campbell Swinton, an electrical engineer, who played an important role in the technical development of radiology, and who set up his own radiographic consulting rooms. He had read the account of the discovery in his morning paper and produced X-rays that same day, possibly the first in England to do so. Photo-graphers and pharmacists hoped to make radiography a profitable side-line, but the

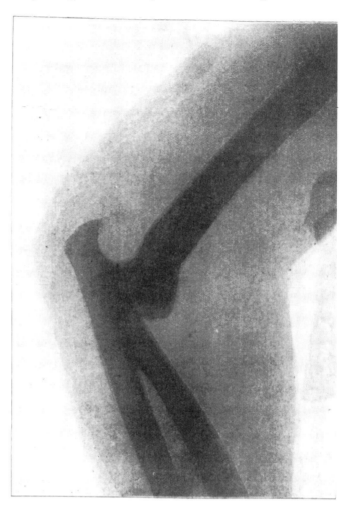

2.5 A case of dislocation of the elbow (*British Medical Journal* 30 May 1896).

capital expense was high, the commitment was time-consuming and most rejected it.

The instrument makers A.E. Dean, Newton and Company and W. Watson and Son were established before 1896, and took advantage of the new discovery not only to expand their range of equipment, but also to demonstrate its use to the medical operators and in some instances to act as radiographers. Several small firms joined them, for example J.H. Montague 'Surgical Instrument Maker and Cutler' [2.6].

Robert Jones was one of the many doctors who realized the possible application of radiography to his own speciality but did not practise it himself. Those who took up the subject were usually at the start of their careers and several, like Macintyre, Dawson Turner of Edinburgh and Mackenzie Davidson of Aberdeen, had a predilection for science or engineering. Thurstan Holland was an exception, learning, as he admitted, by trial and error. Some doctors, notably John Hall-Edwards, were sufficiently confident in their scientific training to emulate Röntgen's experiments on the basis of published reports. He located a needle embedded in a woman's hand on 14 February which was removed the next day. Soon he was able to set up his own radiological practice.

Some teaching hospitals, Charing Cross, the London, St Bartholomew's and Glasgow Royal Infirmary, for example, had already established electrical departments by 1896. Their medical staff, including Hedley and Lewis Jones, and their lay assistants had the skills and most of the apparatus needed for X-ray production. When they heard about the discovery they soon

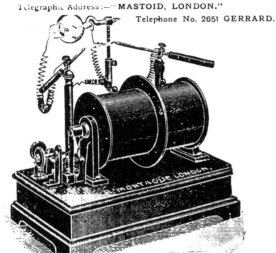
2.6 Advertisement from *The Medical Annual* for 'Rontgen's X-rays' apparatus.

acquired the necessary evacuated glass tubes with electrodes.

By the end of 1896 much had changed. The professors withdrew from practical diagnostic work to concentrate on theoretical problems, though some continued their medical connection in an advisory capacity. The scientific amateurs, with a few exceptions, found radiography too expensive and time-consuming, as did the photographers and pharmacists. Electrical engineers and instrument-makers grew in importance. Medical radiologists started to make an impact, but their numbers were still very small.

The Development of Diagnostic Radiology

The development of diagnostic radiology has resulted from a fruitful interaction between doctors, radiographers, physicists and equipment manufacturers. The production of new apparatus has stimulated the introduction of new techniques and clinical needs have in their turn stimulated new developments in equipment.

The field of diagnostic radiology is now so large that many areas cannot be mentioned in a short review.

Many hospitals obtained X-ray apparatus shortly following the discovery of the new rays by Röntgen in 1895. Many of the pioneers were physicists, photographers and general practitioners. For example, at the London Hospital experiments were undertaken by a physician, Dr Page and a surgeon, Mr Harold Barnard. The initial interest was centred around a photo-graphic club within the hospital. Ernest Harnack who was clerk to the registrars volunteered his services as a radiographer and the first radiograph of a needle in a foot was made early in 1896 [3.1]. Peripheral radiography was not a problem where the body part was thin. Radiography of the trunk was to prove technically more demanding and the shadows produced were much more difficult to interpret. Harnack had three assistants, Reginald Blackall, Ernest Wilson and Harold Suggars. Wilson joined in 1898 to help with the X-ray work and to perform clinical photography. He developed signs of skin damage within a few months and by 1903 they all had radiation injuries. Wilson died of his injuries in 1911 and took a series of photographs of his hands showing progressive bony damage. Harnack ultimately had both arms amputated. Suggars

3.1 The first radiograph taken at the London (now the Royal London) Hospital, January 1896. A needle in a foot.

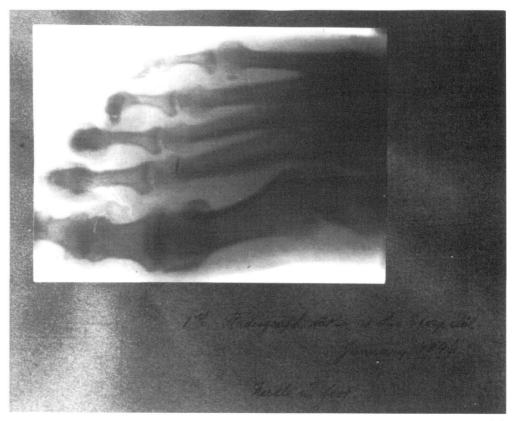

and Blackall worked for longer and helped to establish the College of Radiographers.

The cause of many of the early injuries was the use of fluoroscopy, especially with the cryptoscope which was a hand-held covered fluorescent screen [3.2], and the absence of protection around the screen and the X-ray tube [3.3]. The low power of the apparatus made radiography difficult, particularly of thicker parts. There was also the common practice of using the operator's hand to test the apparatus. In 1921 William Ironside Bruce who was a radiologist at Charing Cross Hospital and the Hospital for Sick Children at Great Ormond Street died of radiation induced injuries. His death sent an immediate shock through the medical community and shortly after the British X-Ray and Radium Protection Committee came into being. This group finally disbanded in 1952.

Ironside Bruce, Reginald Blackall and Ernest Wilson were among the 14 British names on the martyr's memorial in the grounds of St Georges Hospital, Hamburg [3.4]. The name of Ernest Harnack was added in the 1950s.

Chest radiology

The initial apparatus was of low power and therefore fluoroscopy was superior to radio-graphy. In 1896 a chest plate of a girl aged 10 years taken at St Thomas's Hospital took 30 minutes to expose. The initial workers used fluoroscopy almost exclusively, often with the hooded fluorescent screen. It was only with the development of higher-powered apparatus with large induction coils and electrolytic interrupters that instantaneous radiography could be developed. By 1905 better quality films could be obtained. There was also a cultural change needed amongst physicians who initially found it hard to accept that a lesion could exist when it was not clinically apparent and could only be demonstrated radiographically.

The first English book on chest radiology was produced by Hugh Walsham and G.H. Orton in 1905. The initial films were of rather poor quality but they were of diagnostic value enabling, for example the drainage of a pneumothorax under X-ray control by John Fawcett at Guys Hospital in 1907. It is now difficult to imagine the management of chest disease without the benefit of chest radiography.

Additional techniques were gradually added. Although earlier workers had used various contrast agents in the bronchial tree it was Sickard and Forestier in the early 1920s who injected a mixture of iodine and poppy seed oil (lipiodol) and enabled the production of good

3.2 Mode of action of the cryptoscope: D, focus tube; A, body casting shadow on B, fluorescent screen which is seen by the eye at C. *British Medical Journal*, April 1896.

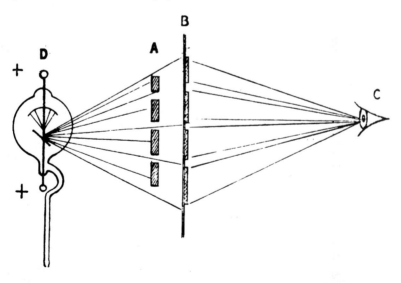

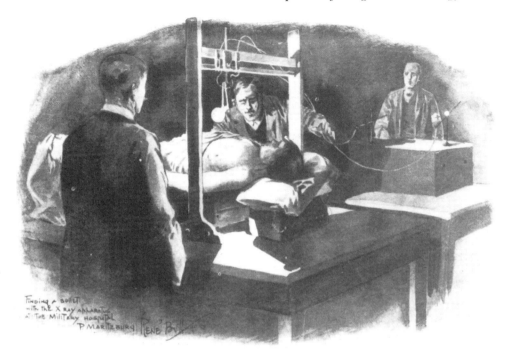

3.3 Finding a bullet with the X-ray apparatus, Pietermartzburg 1899. Note the lack of protection of the tube and the operators.

3.4 The Martyrs Memorial, St Georges Hospital, Hamburg.

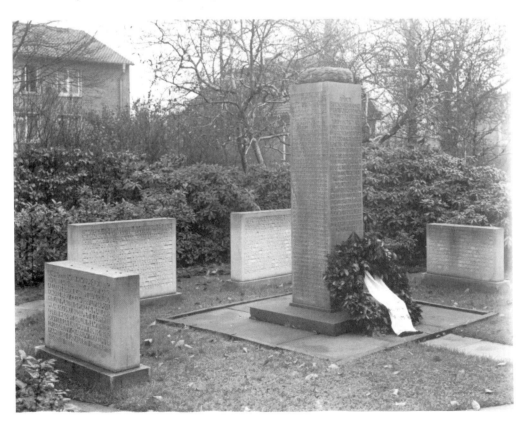

quality bronchography. The use of plain tomography was invented in the 1930s by Bernard Ziedses des Plantes and popularized in the UK by Edward Wing Twining of Manchester. Plain tomography continues to this day although the introduction of CT scanning has considerably reduced the number of indications. There is now a generation of radiologists and radiographers who are unfamiliar with the older techniques of bronchography and tomography which were once so commonly performed.

The techniques used reflected the pathology encountered, bronchiectasis, tuberculosis, lung abscess and empyema being common in the earlier years of this century. Fluoroscopy was extensively used in the management of TB not only to assist in diagnosis but also in the performance of artificial pneumothorax. Dedicated chest fluoroscopic apparatus was used in many chest clinics. In a similar way to the current use of screening mammography, the introduction of mobile miniature-film apparatus in the 1930s by Russell Reynolds and Watsons Ltd enabled the development of mass radiography for the early diagnosis of pulmonary TB. This became particularly important when effective drug treatments were introduced in the 1950s. The apparatus for miniature radiography has gradually been taken out of use and now only few units survive.

The initial anatomical understanding of radiographs was imperfect and considerable work was needed to help sort out the often confusing shadows. In the UK, Sir Thomas Lodge worked on the pulmonary vessels, Lord Brock on bronchial anatomy and George Simon on the lung parenchyma. Lord Brock published his *The Anatomy of the Bronchial Tree* in 1947 and in 1956 the first edition of the influential *The Principles of Chest Radiograph* by George Simon appeared. George Simon closely cooperated with the pathologist Lynne Reid in a series of classic papers on lung pathology. In 1960 Ben Felson produced his *Fundamentals of Chest Radiology*, a classic of medical communication. In 1970 the comprehensive *Diagnosis of Diseases of the Chest* by Fraser and Paré appeared. Peter Kerley worked on bronchial carcinoma and linear shadows (Kerley lines).

The introduction of safe intravascular agents enabled the angiographic demonstration of pulmonary vessels. More recently nuclear medicine, computed tomographic (CT) scanning and magnetic resonance imaging (MRI) have been introduced. These techniques enable detailed anatomy to be demonstrated non-invasively. Pulmonary secondary deposits were first demonstrated on CT by Louis Kreel in 1976. In 1955 there was the first use of a radioactive tracer in the lungs with the introduction of Xenon-133 and external counting. In 1964 pulmonary blood flow was demonstrated using albumen particles labelled with Iodine-131 and in 1975 Fanzio and Jones described the use of Krypton 81M for lung ventilation scanning. The plain radiograph remains central and is being developed by the use of digital computer radiography and other techniques. Modern techniques enable the non-invasive investigation of conditions previously requiring complex and often surgical procedures. Percutaneous biopsy techniques have been introduced for pulmonary and pleural masses and angiography is used for both diagnostic and therapeutic procedures.

The abdomen

The difficulty of visualizing the abdominal organs was related to the thickness and density of the structures involved. As already indicated radiography was difficult because of the low power of the apparatus used. Compression devices were used but because of the lack of contrast in the tissues contrast material had to be introduced. A major initial problem was the extent of new anatomical knowledge required and the identification of normal variants. A landmark was the publication by Köhler in 1910 of the first edition of his classic book on normal variants. To distinguish calcified glands, biliary, renal bladder and phleboliths could be a major problem [3.5]. In the renal tract Harry Fenwick of the London Hospital introduced ureteric bougies to identify the course of the ureters and retrograde studies with contrast material such as collargol soon followed. Intravascular contrast agents were introduced in the 1930s and transformed the examination.

Liquid contrast was introduced into the stomach as the bismuth meal and later using the less toxic barium sulphate. The opaque meal was developed in Vienna in 1904 by Reider and popularized in the UK by workers such as A.E. Barclay and

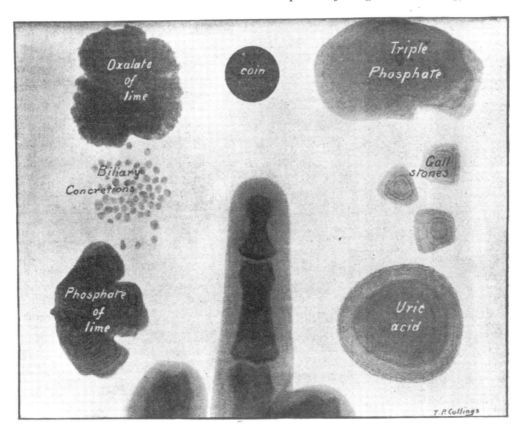

3.5 The relative opacity of calculi, *British Medical Journal* April 1896.

Sebastian Gilbert Scott. Scott's apparatus is illustrated in [3.6]. Rectally administered the colon could be filled by bismuth to assist in the diagnosis of large bowel disease.

The lack of contrast of the unopacified biliary tract was a difficulty until the development of iodine-containing oral contrast agents introduced as the Graham test in 1924. Direct opacification of the gallbladder and biliary tree by large-needle cholangiography was introduced experimentally in 1920 but was dangerous. The modern development of fine needles has allowed the safe performance of many biliary procedures, both for diagnosis and also for treatment of calculi and strictures. The technique of drainage of a biliary obstruction is now often done as a team effort between radiologist and endoscopist.

Use of techniques

In modern radiological practice it is not possible to consider techniques in isolation. An integrated approach is needed with the various techniques used as appropriate. Often it is better for complex procedures to be used early in an investigation since a diagnosis may be reached quickly with minimum inconvenience and risk to the patient. In recent years the widespread use of percutaneous biopsy techniques and ultrasound and CT scanning have considerably reduced the need for exploratory surgery. In many departments now, ultrasound is the most commonly performed procedure after the plain film. There have been many changes in medicine which influence radiological practice. For example, the increasing use of endoscopy has considerably reduced the need for barium meals. There has been a marked trend in recent years towards the management of patients either as outpatients or day cases. Recent developments in diagnostic imaging have considerably facilitated this trend with considerably less disruption of the patient's life.

Until the 1980s the techniques needed to store reports and films had changed little since the

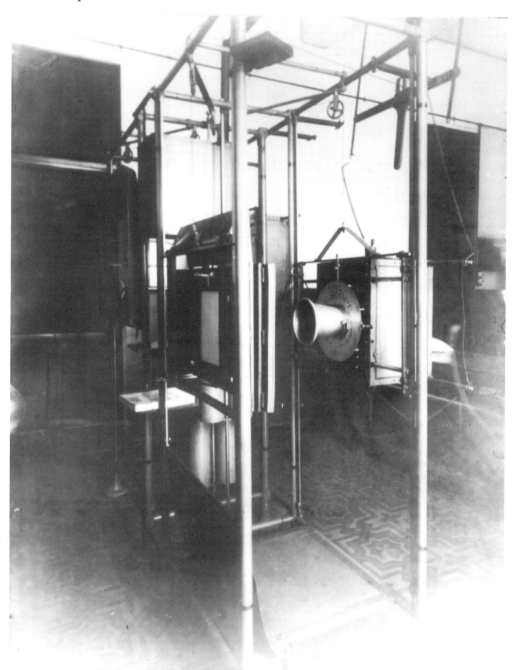

3.6 Apparatus used by Sebastian Gilbert Scott at the London Hospital, 1921.

1920s. Modern digital technology is transforming radiology departments by the introduction of computer management systems improving both communication and digital image storage. This last technique will dramatically alter the use of images with radiological studies being transferred via links between different institutions and offices. The last 100 years has produced many changes and the next 100 will be even more dramatic.

History of Neuroradiology

It is appropriate that in this centenary celebration of the discovery of X-rays by Röntgen in 1895 that we look back upon the history of neuroradiology and of the illustrious careers and achievements of earlier pioneers. The achievements, which have been prodigious, have had major repercussions not just in clinical neurosciences but indeed in some other clinical specialties also. The achievements of the last 100 years are all the more glittering when one contrasts these with the very limited diagnostic means which were available to earlier physicians and surgeons. Indeed in earlier times even dreams were accepted as being a valid means of diagnosis. The reality of diagnostic dreams was accepted by physicians from Hippocrates to Galen. It is incredible that such superstitious beliefs were so tenaciously held and how late have been the developments of more scientific diagnostic radiological studies. It was only in July 1939 that the first Symposium Neuroradiologicum was held in Antwerp.

The first 65 years of the history of neuroradiology were described in the Presidential address delivered by Dr James Bull at the British Institute of Radiology on 20 October 1960. Much of the information given in this brief resume is obtained from his paper. In the audience on that occasion were several who had lived through the discovery of X-rays and the early development of diagnostic radiology.

Dr Bull's interest in the early history of radiology is also demonstrated in his choice of subject for his MacKenzie Davidson Memorial Lecture on 17 February 1972 some twelve years later, which was titled 'Neuroradiology's debt to Becquerel'. In 1896, only a few months after Röntgen's discovery, one of the earliest diagnostic radiologists working in Birmingham (Major Hall-Edwards) used X-rays for the localization of a foreign body. In the Boer War of 1898, Major Hall-Edwards used his localization device for identification of shrapnel fragments. The technique was also used intracranial foreign bodies. It is, however, Arthur Schuller born in Brun in 1874 who is regarded as the father of neuroradiology [4.1].

In 1912 Schuller published a textbook on radiology of the skull. He pointed out the value of identifying the calcified pineal gland. He also categorized many types of benign and malignant intracranial calcification. He even devised a transphenoidal approach for the treatment of pituitary tumours. In 1938 he was forced to flee Hitler's Austria and settled in Melbourne. Schuller, who is described as a charming and helpful colleague, nevertheless had a very sad life. His two sons died in concentration camps.

In 24 November 1912 a middle-aged American was admitted following a head injury to a New York hospital under the care of Dr W. H. Luckett. Radiographs were performed by W. H. Stewart

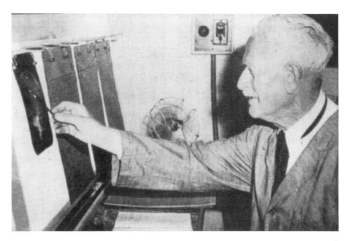

4.1 Arthur Schuller, the father of neuroradiology.

who detected a fracture in the posterior wall of the frontal sinus. The patient who was treated conservatively was later discharged but admitted three weeks later having suffered a relapse. Subsequent skull X-ray showed the cerebral ventricles to be enormously dilated by what was thought to be air or gas [4.2]. Following this, Dr Luckett operated and tapped one of the ventricles, releasing air or gas. The patient died three days later (these were early days for neurosurgery too). Autopsy confirmed a fracture of the posterior wall of the frontal sinus with a depressed bone fragment. The brain immediately upon its removal, was placed under water and bubbles emerged through a tear in the base of the frontal lobe. This tear was shown to communicate with the frontal horn of the lateral ventricle. Dandy in 1918 developed the technique of air ventriculography and shortly afterwards in 1919 introduced air encephalography. He also predicted air myelography but did not follow this up until 1925 by which time Sicard and Forestier in Paris had used Lipiodol in the localisation of spinal blocks.

Then as now, neurosurgeons still required ever improving diagnostic techniques. Demonstration of the arterial supply of the brain was achieved by Egas Moniz a Portuguese neurologist born in 1874 and trained under Babinski in Paris. In 1919 he fought a duel. Fortunately he survived and in the middle of the 1920's described the brain as 'the dark continent normally mute to X-rays'. He thought it might be possible to solve this problem by the intravenous injection of large quantities of elements with relatively high atomic numbers in the hope that tumours and other masses would accept the injected material and thus cast a shadow on a radiograph. He was much influenced in this opinion by Graham and Cole who in 1924 outlined the gallbladder by injecting the sodium salt of tetrabromophenolthphalein intravenously. This technique depended upon the excretion of the salt by the liver and its concentration in the gallbladder. No comparable physiological principle existed in the brain and Moniz's ill-founded attempts failed, when in 1927 he gave large quantities intravenously and by mouth of lithium and strontium bromide. Despite this mistaken belief, Moniz went on to the great discovery of cerebral arteriography [4.3], by using a 25% sodium iodide solution to opacify blood vessels supplying the brain. In his ninth case of arterial injection of 5ml 25% soldium iodide good views of the carotid artery and its branches were achieved. One patient died 8 hours after this procedure. Difficulties would be experienced to-day obtaining ethical committee approval but this experience certainly exemplifies Moniz's great determination and persistence.

Another great name from these early days of neuroradiology is Erik Lysholm who was born in 1891 and became neuroradiologist at the Serafimer Hospital in Stockholm. In 1925 he published a paper on radiography of the petrous bone and in 1936 the monumental *Das Ventrikulogram*. Lysholm, together with the engineer Schonander, developed the first dedicated skull X-ray table [4.4]. This device employed the principle of moving an X-ray table around an imaginary sphere with the central ray always directed towards the centre of the sphere. The angles of rotation of the X-ray tube were related to anatomical reference lines of the skull. Lysholm in Sweden and two other radiologists in the UK and USA worked on the manipulation of air within the ventricular system. These others were Edward Wing Twining [4.5] in Manchester and Cornelius Dyke in New York. Twining made an ingenious model of the ventricular system using a small quantity of

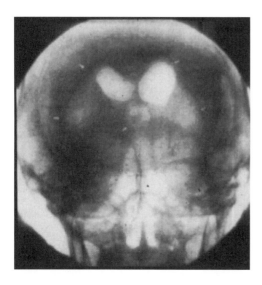

4.2 Accidental observation of air in the cerebral ventricles by W. H. Luckett in 1912.

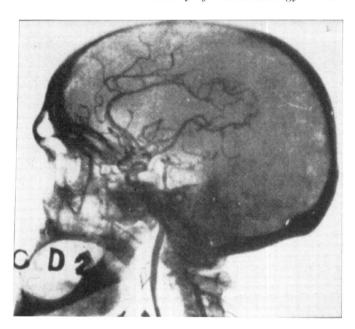

4.3 Early cerebral angiogram by
Egas Moniz in 1927.

mercury which could then be inversely projected
as a lantern slide to illustrate the principles of air
encephalography. Using this model it could be
shown how a gas could be manipulated
throughout the complex ventricular system.

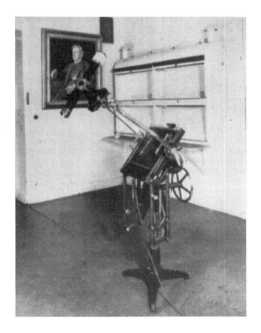

4.4 Lysholm-Schonander skull table developed in
1931. Note the Gosta Forschell portrait. Gosta
Forschell was the father of Swedish radiology.

This model is still in existence. Cornelius Dyke,
born in 1900, together with Davidoff the neuro-
surgeon, published *The Normal Encephalogram*
in 1937. This partnership studied the radiology
of the cisterns and subarachnoid CSF pathways

During the subsequent 35 years, a process of
consolidation occurred with improvements in
equipment as well as in vascular contrast agents.
Isotope brain imaging was the next major
development, when in 1948 Moore attempted
to define cerebral tumours more precisely. It
was known that some tumours e.g. gliomas took
up fluorescein selectively. In ultraviolet light
such tumours stood out, reflecting a different
colour. Moore established at craniotomy with
the brain cortex exposed, that a beam of UV
light shone upon glioma, yielded a yellowish
colour whilst the surrounding normal brain
had a blue/grey colouration. The brilliant step
which Moore then took was to tag a radioactive
substance on to the fluorescein so that he
might be able to identify the tumour using a
Geiger counter. This radioactive dye-iodofluor-
escein he injected intravenously, in exactly the
same way that he had injected fluorescein alone.
He successfully detected gamma rays not only
from gliomas but also from other tumours. In
the following years significant improvements
took place in detector systems and also in
radiopharmaceuticals.

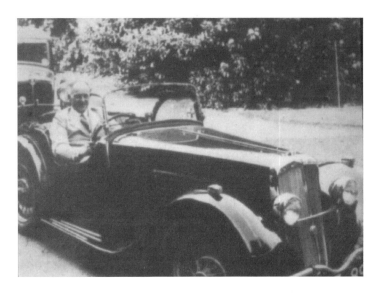

4.5 Edward Wing Twining.

The next major leap was in 1972 when computerized axial tomography scanning was described by Ambrose and Hounsfield at the British Institute of Radiology. Until then X-ray techniques had relied on X-ray film as the recording medium and the presentation of 3D

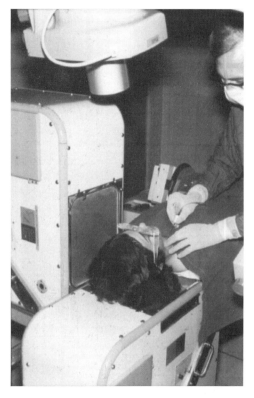

4.6 Percutaneous carotid angiogram in the 1950s. The patient is wearing protective lead spectades.

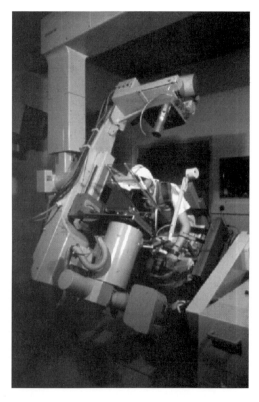

4.7 Air encephalography using a Murier 3 orbiting skull unit in the 1960s.

information on a 2D film. This is not of course the most efficient means of detecting X-rays.

Oldendorf in 1961 performed experiments to display the internal structure of complex objects using an isotope source of radiation. Reconstruction facilities were not then fully developed to take further advantage of this approach. Hounsfield using a more efficient detector system, directed the X-ray beam—collimated—at a series of transverse slices which were irradiated via their edges. The numerical data generated was then processed using a computer and displayed as a black and white image.

These first generation, translate/rotate CT scanners [4.7] were extremely slow by modern standards but were revolutionary in concept and changed neuroradiological practice. Despite their original 80×80 matrix, restrictive water bag and long scan and reconstruction times (6 images in 35 minutes) the 'dark continent' was finally revealed. This technique significantly reduced the need for angiography. Percutaneous carotid and vertebral angiography [4.6] were replaced by femoral artery catheter techniques described first by Seldinger in 1953. Ventriculography and air encephalography [4.7] were all but abandoned.

Over the last decade we have seen the application of magnetic resonance imaging (MRI), Doppler ultrasound and interventional neuroradiological techniques which have maintained the momentum for change initiated by Hounsfield and Ambrose. Functional MRI and spectroscopy are now becoming available as clinical tools. We have yet to see these exciting new techniques realise their full potential. Over the last quarter of a century, the considerable achievements of neuroradiology have far exceeded the most crazed diagnostic dreams. We can be confident that with the ever increasing range of neuroradiology, the future will be just as dazzling.

5

Interventional Radiology

In the last three decades diagnostic radiologists have become increasingly involved in the active management of patients, with the development of percutaneous techniques not only for diagnosis but also for treatment. Interventional procedures under the guidance of fluoroscopy, ultrasound or computed tomography have, in many instances, replaced open operations by surgeons under general anaesthesia, resulting in lower morbidity, earlier mobilization and reduced hospital stay. Close co-operation between radiologists and clinicians is essential to optimize patient management.

Many pioneers and innovators have contributed to the development of interventional radiology, which has its roots in angiography. Angiography was developed in the late 1920s by a brilliant group of Portuguese experimental and clinical investigators. Cerebral angiography was introduced in 1927 by Moniz, a distinguished politician and Professor of Neurology and Psychiatry at Lisbon University, and translumbar aortography in 1929 by dos Santos. Another milestone of seminal importance also occurred in 1929 when Forssmann, in Berlin, carried out the first catheterization of the human right heart (his own!), using a compliant urethral catheter.

A giant leap forwards in the development of angiography occurred in 1953, when the technique of percutaneous catheterization was published. Seldinger's elegant innovation revolutionized arteriography, greatly expanding its diagnostic capabilities. Other factors contributing to the development of angiography include the introduction of conventional contrast media in the mid 1950s, the development of selective catheterization techniques, the construction of radio-opaque and torque-control catheters, innovations in guide wire technology, the use of pressure injectors, and advances in X-ray tube design and image recording systems.

The birth of interventional radiology occurred early in 1963, when Dotter, using Seldinger's technique, passed a catheter percutaneously through an occluded iliac artery whilst undertaking retrograde abdominal aortography in a patient with diminished femoral pulsation. This initial inadvertent transluminal recanalization led Dotter to conceive the idea that atherosclerotic obstruction could be relieved by catheter techniques. He developed a co-axial catheter system for dilating arterial lesions in the legs but transluminal dilatation only gained widespread acceptance following the introduction of noncompliant balloons by Grüntzig in 1974. Later that decade Grüntzig reported dilatating renal and coronary arteries stenoses using small co-axial balloons introduced through guiding catheters. The advent of percutaneous transluminal angioplasty revolutionized the management of patients with occlusive arterial disease and the range of lesions amenable to treatment by angioplasty has since been greatly extended by advances in balloon technology and guide wire construction. Veins can be dilated as can stenotic heart valves, and balloons are also used in the management of a variety of non-vascular obstructions which, will be mentioned later.

The 1970s saw the emergence of another interventional catheter procedure that of therapeutic embolization. This percutaneous method of vascular occlusion can be used in a variety of clinical situations including the control of haemorrhage (including postbiopsy bleeding), the treatment of abnormal vascular communications, the occlusion of aneurysms, the reduction of tumour vascularity prior to surgery and the ablation of functioning endocrine tumours. In the venous system, embolization can be used to occlude varicoceles and, transhepatically, to obliterate oesophageal varices. Many different substances have been used to effect vascular occlusion, including particulate materials, liquid tissue adhesives, and mechanical devices such as steel coils and detachable balloons.

Other mechanical devices can be introduced into the body using interventional techniques. Vena caval filters for pulmonary embolism prophylaxis were first described in the late 1960s but they had to be inserted through a surgical venotomy. The 1980s saw the development of caval filters with low profile introducing sheaths, allowing percutaneous insertion, and thus greatly facilitating the use of these devices. The 1980s also saw the clinical application of metallic stents, first reported in the experimental model by Dotter in 1969, and a number of different types, all expensive, are currently under evaluation. In the vascular system they have been used as an adjunct or alternative to conventional percutaneous transluminal angioplasty, to relieve superior vena caval obstruction, to effect transhepatic portal-systemic shunts, and, more recently, in endovascular grafting for the treatment of abdominal aortic aneurysms. The use of stents in non-vascular situations is discussed below.

Arterial catheterization techniques have been developed for the local infusion of drugs, including thrombolytic agents (first undertaken in 1971) and chemotherapeutic substances. More recently, methods have been devised for the percutaneous placement of permanent catheters and ports under local anaesthesia for the intravenous administration of various types of medication.

Percutaneous extraction of an intravascular foreign body was first reported in 1964 and since that time various retrieval devices have been introduced. Other percutaneous catheter extraction techniques include thromboembolectomy and atherectomy.

The development of image-guided needle techniques for obtaining tissue samples for cytological and/or histological diagnosis has been a great advance in patient management, obviating the need for open biopsy in most cases. A natural progression was the development of percutaneous drainage procedures, now widely used to treat abscesses and other types of fluid collection in many parts of the body.

Percutaneous neurological interventional procedures include embolization of congenital arteriovenous malformations, occlusion of cerebral aneurysms and carotico-cavernous fistulae [5.1], and percutaneous transluminal angioplasty of arch, carotid, vertebral and even intracerebral arteries.

In the chest, interventional techniques include percutaneous biopsy of lung and mediastinal masses, embolization of congenital arteriovenous malformations, embolization of bronchial arteries for controlling recurrent or massive haemoptysis, stenting of tracheobronchial stenoses, recanalization of superior

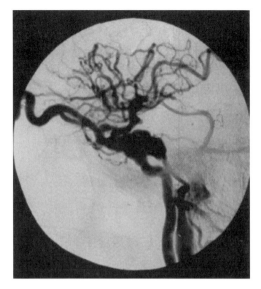

(a)

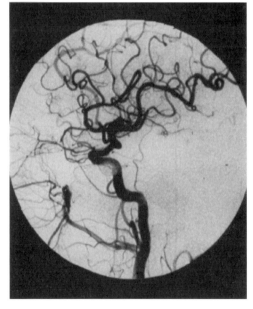

(b)

5.1 Occlusion of carotico-cavernous fistula with 8 mm detachable latex balloon:
(a) lateral angiogram before occlusion showing early venous filling;
(b) after occlusion of the fistula no venous filling is seen.
(Courtesy of Dr B. Kendall)

vena caval obstruction, and needle aspiration or catheter drainage of pleural and mediastinal fluid collections. Cardiac percutaneous catheter interventions include coronary angioplasty, coronary stenting, balloon valvuloplasty, closure of congenital cardiovascular defects, endomyocardial biopsy, and the catheter ablation of arrhythmias.

Percutaneous biliary procedures commenced in the 1930s in Asia with drainage of liver abscesses. In the 1970s they were refined with the introduction of the fine bore 'Chiba' needle enabling bile ducts of whatever size to be entered in virtually 100% of patients, so providing diagnostic cholangiograms. The use of percutaneously introduced external or combined external/internal drainage catheters to treat infected or obstructed bile ducts quickly followed. A natural progression of this was to employ balloon catheters to dilate strictures or stents to bridge obstructions. In the past decade, the use of small diameter catheters and larger (up to 12 mm) diameter expanding metal stents have both improved treatment choice for clinicians and patients, and greatly lowered the complication rates associated with a transhepatic approach. Other biliary interventional procedures include percutaneous cholecystostomy under ultrasound guidance as an alternative to surgical cholecystostomy in patients requiring emergency treatment for acute cholecystitis, and the removal of gallstones through T-tube tracks. Besides percutaneous biopsy, other hepatic interventional procedures include embolization,

transcatheter chemotherapy, transjugular intrahepatic portosystemic stent shunts (TIPSS) [5.2], and laser ablation of tumours. Pancreatic masses can be biopsied safely under image-guidance and pancreatic pseudocysts are amenable to percutaneous drainage, as are subphrenic abscesses and other intra-abdominal fluid collections.

Therapeutic image-guided procedures of the kidney commenced in 1952 with diagnostic puncture of cysts and tumours. In the 1980s interventional uroradiology increased in volume and variety. Percutaneous nephrostomy, stent placement, stone removal, dilatation of arterial stenoses in native [5.3] and transplant kidneys, and embolization of arteriovenous fistulae (some iatrogenic) have become standard procedures. As in many other body regions, it is both sensible and safe to perform renal biopsy under some form of imaging guidance. The development of transrectal ultrasound has enabled prostatic biopsy to be carried out accurately.

Interventional techniques have also been applied to other organ stems. In the gastrointestinal tract, oesophageal dilatation, stent placement and percutaneous gastrostomy deserve special mention. In the musculoskeletal system, image-guided percutaneous biopsy is a common procedure in the investigation of focal

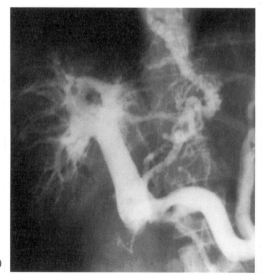

(a)

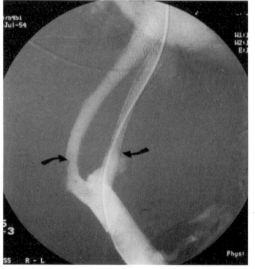

5.2 TIPS shunt between hepatic and portal vein using two expandable stainless steel 'Wallstents' to lower portal hypertension.
(a) Planning portal venogram with variceal filling.

(b) Stents (arrowed) *in situ* with no variceal filling and shunting of blood to the lower-pressure systemic venous system.

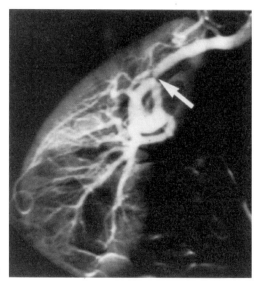

(a)

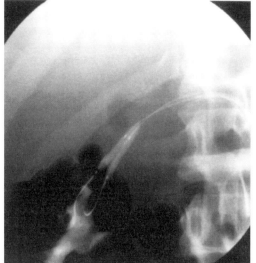

(b)

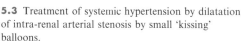

5.3 Treatment of systemic hypertension by dilatation of intra-renal arterial stenosis by small 'kissing' balloons.
(a) Angiogram before angioplasty showing stenosis (arrowed).
(b) 'Kissing' balloons dilating stenosis.
(c) Angiogram after angioplasty showing abolition of stenosis.
(Courtesy of Dr R. Edwards)

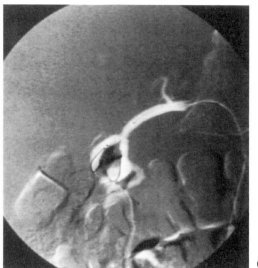

(c)

bone lesions and suspected intervertebral disc infection. Therapeutic interventional procedures can be used in the management of both benign and malignant bone tumours, and to treat intervertebral disc protrusion. Interventional procedures also have a very important role in the localization and biopsy of breast lesions, and have been used in the treatment of infertility.

Interventional radiology is in a continuing state of evolution. This innovative specialty led to the concept of minimally invasive therapy, an operative approach developed in the last few years that is predicted to revolutionize all forms of conventional surgery in the coming decades.

Apparatus in Diagnostic Radiology

Before the discovery

To enable Röntgen to make his great discovery of X-rays a century ago, three fields of physics needed to come together in fairly advanced state of development. First, the production of vacuum pumps and the study of their vacuum. Second, the study of electricity leading to Faraday's brilliant work on electromagnetic induction, and consequently to the production of a reliable source of high tension. Third, the intensive study of discharge phenomena and ultimately cathode rays, which constructed the foundations of not only X-ray tubes, but electronic valves, image intensifiers and cathode ray monitors. In the seventeenth century Guericke, and a little latter Hauksbee, not only developed the first vacuum pump but also studied the production of electrical discharges *in vacuo*.

Michael Faraday's discovery of electro-magnetic induction lead to the development of induction coils, without which the reliable production of kilovoltage necessary to produce X-radiation would have been unobtainable. Towards the end of the 19th century both Sir William Crookes and Johan Hittorf were examining the properties of cathode rays, Crookes had even developed a 45° target and must unbeknown to him have produced X-rays. Thus the stage was set for Röntgen's momentous discovery.

The early equipment

The apparatus that Röntgen used to discover the existence of X-rays consisted of a partially evacuated pear-shaped Hittorf-Crookes tube, using a Ruhmkorff induction coil to produce the electrical discharge. Figure 6.1 shows the Russell Reynolds X-ray equipment of 1896 with the basically similar components.

The development of the modern X-ray tube

The original X-ray tube [6.2] consisted of a flat aluminium cathod with the anode connection in

a side arm off the glass pear; the X-rays were produced by interaction with the glass.

These tubes were very unreliable often only lasting a few exposures.

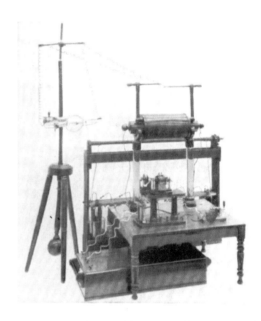

6.1 The Russell Reynolds X-ray equipment (1896–7).

Many designs of these so called, 'gas tubes' were introduced between 1895 and 1913 when the Coolidge tube made it's appearance. They

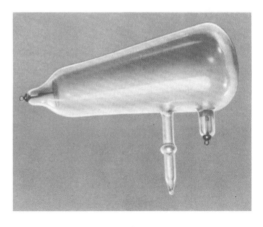

6.2 A Crookes' tube used by Röntgen to produce the first known X-rays.

were not designed to work in a vacuum, and often contained heavy extra electrodes called anti-kathodes which were heated, and acted as a sponge, absorbing and releasing the residual gas which constituted the vehicle for exciting the tube.

W.D. Coolidge's introduction of the hot cathode tube in 1913 was one of the biggest turning points in the diagnostic application of X-rays. Thermionic emission had been observed as early as th 18th Century, and was employed in the valve invented by Thomas Eddison in 1883, but it was not until the advent of the separately heated tungsten filament of Coolidge's tube that the current and voltage could be independently controlled. Operating at 100 kV and 200 mamp maximum this tube could produce exposures undreamed of the year before. The next major steps in X-ray tube design were introduced by the Dutch engineer A. Bouwers. Working for Philips, he introduced in 1924 the Metalix tube which was cylindrical in shape and surrounded by chrome-iron alloy fused to the glass. Around this was situated a lead collar, thus creating the first fully protected insert. A year later Bouwers was also credited with the introduction of the first functional tungsten rotating anode tube.

Since Bouwers' day tubes have shown continual refinement with such changes as Goetze's introduction of line focus, three-phase high-speed rotation, and the use of a grid bias to the cathode cup for rapid serial switching. Figure 6.3 shows

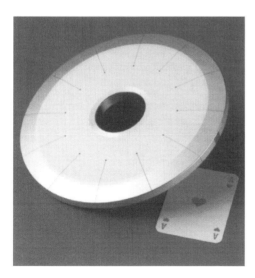

6.3 The Philips MRC-200 tube for digital cardiac imaging.

the anode from a Maximum Rotalix Ceramic MRC-200 which is directly liquid cooled, and the absence of ball-bearings provides rotation without a sound. It represents the most advanced X-ray tube now available with heat storage capacity of 2,400,000 heat units.

Plates, screens and fluoroscopes

It can be said that fluoroscopy outdated radiography, just, because Röntgen must have first viewed his hand on the barium-platinocyanide screen before producing the first radiograph of Frau Röntgen's hand. However for that first radiograph to be possible the photographic industry had been through a century of progress in emulsions, and both plates and film would have been available in 1895. In 1896 Thomas Edison published a list of 72 substances which were known to fluoresce under X-ray excitation. He demonstrated that calcium tungstate was several times better than platino barium cyanide, but it was not until about 1914 that new phosphors such as cadmium tungstate were introduced. Conventional fluoroscopy is old and changed little in principle from the cryptoscope employed in Perugia by Salvioni in 1896, or the more sophisticated screening equipment used in the first half of this century.

Image intensifiers had been first suggested in 1924 by M. C. Teves, but we had to wait until the infrared night-viewing devices of World War II, to allow Westinghouse to introduce them. The early image intensifiers were very large using an image orthicon tube and a Bouwers' concentric lens system. This bulk was much reduced in the 1970s and 1980s but with the new generation of 35 mm metal intensifiers, we seem to have come full circle.

It was soon realized that photographic emulsion alone was not sufficient to produce an optimum photographic effect. The use of intensifying screens with plates and later with film have been with us in the form of calcium tungstate since 1896. These remained paramount until the introduction by the film manufacturers of rare earth screens, previously investigated by Sir William Crookes in 1896, in the 1970s.

X-ray cassettes are now much lighter, being manufactured in plastic with identification windows, and can be handled by the new

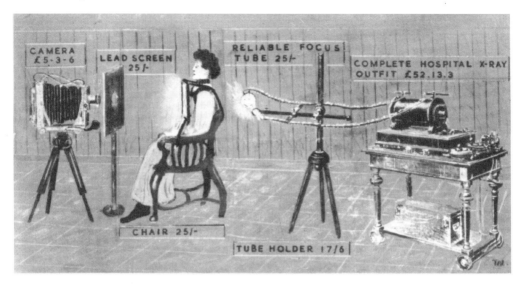

6.4 Photofluorographic equipment, with prices, in 1898.

multi-loaders processing systems now in use. Film is now available with the new improved flat grains with sensitivity to either blue or green spectral emission from the rate earth phosphors.

Photographic processing has moved on from shallow dishes, through deep tank manual development and automatic dunking systems to the sophisticated micro-processor controlled roller processors used in the multi-loaders mentioned above.

6.5 A room in the Whithington Hospital in 1957 showing Watson apparatus and no visible protection at the control panel.

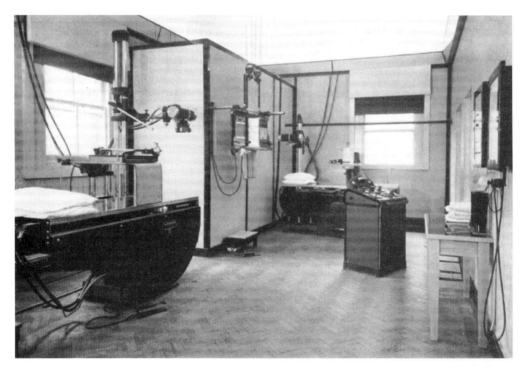

Control of unwanted and secondary radiation

A device which has long been basic to radiography practice is the Potter-Bucky diaphragm. It is surprising to note that the original device was situated at the tube window for the removal of scattered radiation from the tube. It was considerably later that it was moved to its present-day position between the patient and film. In 1913 Dr J. Bucky in Germany introduced a metallic honeycomb device which left a criss-cross pattern on the film. In 1916 Dr H. E. Potter of the USA moved this device during exposure to blue out the pattern. In 1917 it was moved to where it has been ever since between the patient and film. Grid design shows little development with lead slats being still used as the absorbing media. However the interspace material, has changed successively from wood, bakelite and aluminium to the modern wonder material carbon fibre. In the same year G. Holznecht suggested a straight tube between patient and screen to cut out scatter and improve definition when screening, so the use of collimation was also introduced around this time. Cones for beam limitation gave way in the 1940s and 1950s to lead controlled adjustable diaphragms, which were the precursor of the much undervalued light beam diaphragm introduced in the 1960s.

The generation of high voltages

At the end of the nineteenth century the two methods of choice for producing the kilovoltages required were either the induction coil or the Wilmshurst machine. The latter was cheap and on a dry day could be effective, however it's performance was such reduced by damp and dust in the atmosphere. It was not until 1907 that H. C. Snook of Philadelphia introduced the high-tension transformer. Transformers were continually developed until, by about 1940, rectified three-phase units were available, with six diode valve secondary rectification. Developments since 1945 have produced 12 pulse solid state rectification, capacitor discharge mobiles, constant potential units with secondary switching, and solid state interrupter technology. Today's medium-frequency units, with solid state micro chip technology, have drastically reduced the bulk of the electrical components, freeing up space for other activities

Radiological tables

The early X-ray couches were little more than simple tables with either wooden or canvas tops. However they quickly developed for various specialist purposes depending on their requirements. Some had dished tops with a curved Potter-Buckey and others had facilities for fluoroscopy. Tables developed to allow tilt of the table and movement of the table top in various directions. In the 1960s over-couch image intensifiers came into vogue with remote control and 90/90 couch tilt. Units for A/E boasted ceiling suspended tubes, floating-top tables, with self-centring and motor-driven vertical movement. The advent of automatic exposure control dates from 1949 when Franke and Bischoffe produced the original Iontomat at

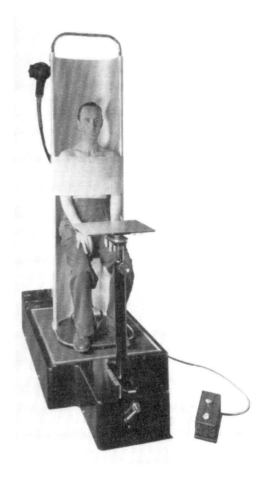

6.6 The Sectograph for horizontal tomography in the 1930s.

Erlangen for Siemens, initially installed within a chest unit, but a year later it was also used for general work.

Tomography

Grossman proposed tomography in 1935, in which linear body section radiography could be carried out on a specially designed table. Conversion kits were supplied to allow multi-use units to be used for linear tomography, but the results were never as good as those obtained with the specially designed table. Also in the mid thirties two pieces of apparatus were built in London to perform erect horizontal body-section fluoroscopy, and transverse body-section radiography. Neither unit was satisfactory, but produced similar, if somewhat blurred, images to CT. B. G. Ziedes des Plantes invented a multi-movement tomographic unit called the Polytome, which was eventually commercially produced in the 1950s by Massiot in France. This unit was highly successful and many are still in use today. The CT scanner came as something of a surprise. It was introduced by

G. Hounsfield of EMI, a previously non radiological firm which completely revolutionized the radiological world. It had jumped a generation in digital and computer controlled development. It is only now that non-tomographic digitised images are being used.

Systems used less at present

The history of radiology has been punctuated by techniques which come in and go out of popularity. Listed here are techniques used less at present but which could regain popularity in the future:

stereography (J. Mackenzie Davidson 1896);
foreign body localization (J. Mackenzie Davidson 1897);
radiographic polaroid system (E. H. Land 1947);
xerography (Xerox Company 1950).

New and future developments

Using television in 1964, analogue images where stored on magnetic video tape and subtraction techniques were carried out for angiographic

6.7 The Philips Integris state-of-the-art digital imaging system.

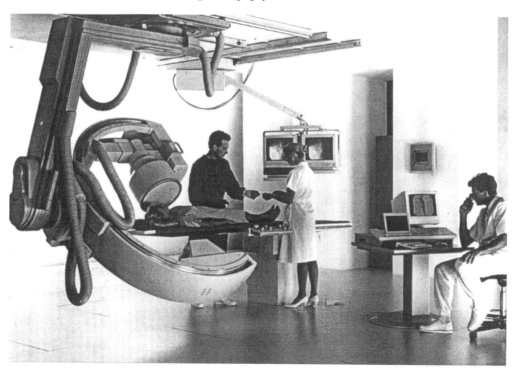

examinations. The technique was not pursued because the results were not acceptable. However with the advent of digital subtraction imaging and also digital spot imaging, and PACS (Picture Archiving and Communication System) the demise of the photographic film has been predicted. Imaging departments today may have digitised images from several mod-

alities queuing up for hard processing on single coated film through laser technology. Plain images can be interrogated by either laser or electrostatic means, to produced a digital image which can be processed later so ensuring a post processing reduced does to the patient, whilst also being capable of transfer worldwide on the electronic information highway.

The Historical Development of Intravascular Radiological Contrast Agents

During Röntgen's original experiments in Würzburg, Germany in November 1895, he demonstrated that substances of high atomic number absorbed his new rays more effectively than did substances of lower atomic number. He documented this on the first human X-ray that of his wife's hand, X-rayed on 22 December 1895, on which her wedding ring is seen to be more radiopaque than the bones or soft tissues.

The first documented use of radiological contrast medium was achieved a few days later in Vienna in early January 1896 when a young physicist, Haschek, and a young physician, Lidenthal, injected a calcium carbonate emulsion into the brachial artery of the severed arm of a cadaver. This first arteriogram was given an exposure time of 57 minutes and was published on 23 January 1896 in *Klinische Wochenschrift*. The first successful visceral angiogram—a renal arteriogram—was probably achieved by Hicks, a physicist at Sheffield University on 6 February 1896 and was published in the *British Medical Journal* on 22 February the same year.

The first clinical human arteriograms and venograms were produced with solutions of strontium bromide and sodium iodide by Berberich and Hirsch in Frankfurt, Germany, and by Brooks in St. Louis, USA in 1923.

Egas Moniz [7.1] in Lisbon, Portugal was enthralled by the success of myelography with lipiodol (discovered by the accidental injection into the subarachnoid space by Sicard and Forestier in Paris in 1921). Moniz was determined to pursue the objective of clinical carotid arteriography for the diagnosis and localization of cerebral tumours. In a long series of animal experiments, he tried lipiodol emulsion, solutions of bromide and iodide salts of sodium, potassium, lithium, strontium and rubidium. His first successful human carotid arteriogram was obtained using a 30% solution of sodium iodide on 27 June 1927 in a young man with a pituitary tumour.

Intravenous urography

Douglas Cameron, a young Minnesota surgeon published in (the *Journal of the American Medical Association*) in 1917, the first use of sodium iodide to produce a urinary cystogram. The Mayo Clinic team of Osborne (syphilologist), Sutherland (radiologist), Scholl (urologist) and Rowntree (physician) published the first scientific paper in JAMA 10 February 1923 on intravenous urography with intravenous sodium iodide (20 g) after the venereologist had noted a cystogram on an abdominal radiograph, in a syphilitic patient being treated with large doses of sodium and potassium iodide. This team produced good intravenous cystograms and modest pyelograms and they related the administered iodide dose to the urinary concentration of iodine.

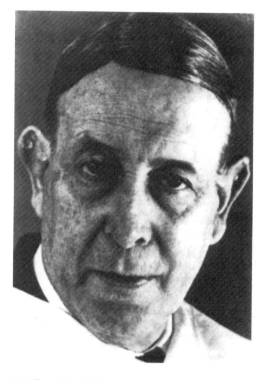

7.1 Egas Moniz (1847–1955)

Attempts to produce a diagnostic quality intravenous urograms (IVUS) were continued by several investigators including Professor von Lichtenberg (Berlin) who in 1905 had introduced retrograde pyelography with Collargol (a colloidal preparation of silver). Hryntschalk of Vienna succeeded in obtaining fairly good calyceal visualization in animals and humans with intravenous injections of Preparation 13, the formula of which he did not disclose. von Lichtenberg was however very despondent of ever achieving diagnostic quality IVUS and 'thought it was an impossible dream' (1927).

Moses Swick (1900–1985 [7.2]) a 1924 graduate of Columbia University, New York, worked at Mount Sinai Hospital, New York where he was awarded a Libman (of Libman-Sack's DLE syndrome) scholarship to study research procedures abroad. He chose to work at Lichtwitz's medical Altona clinic in Hamburg where he studied the therapeutic potential of a series of iodinated products synthesized by Binz and Rath of The Agricultural College in Berlin.

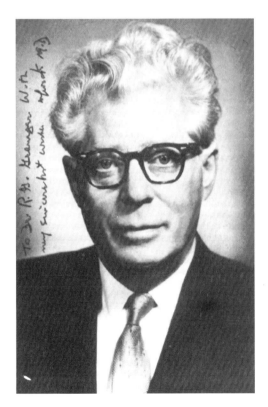

7.2 Moses Swick (1900–1985)

Swick observed that reasonable quality IVUS could be obtained after intravenous injection of some of these products into laboratory animals and so transferred his research to work on urological patients at von Lichtenberg's clinic at St Hedwig's Hospital, Berlin. This was then the largest surgical urological clinical in the world. It was at that clinic in 1929 that Swick succeeded in producing excellent quality diagnostic IVU's in patients using Binz and Rath preparations— Selectan Neutral (a non-ionic mono-iodinated pyridone molecule) and also with the less toxic but more soluble Uroselectan (sodium 5-iodo-2-pyridone N acetate, patent rights awarded to Rath in Berlin on 12 May 1927.)

von Lichtenberg was in America during Swick's development of these superb quality IVUS, and the professor returned to Berlin after receiving Swick's cable. Most unfortunately, a bitter personal confrontation developed between the young inexperienced Swick and the prestigious professor concerning attribution of the successful research and the priority of publication. It was eventually decided with the help of von Salle (editor of *Klinische Wochenschrift*) that the first paper announcing the very important diagnostic discovery should be by Swick alone (1929), immediately followed in the same issue of the journal by a combined paper by von Lichtenberg and Swick on the clinical applications of Uroselectan IVU.

But the tragic and pathetic personal confrontation was only resolved 36 years later when Marshall, Professor of Urological Surgery in New York conducted a very detailed assessment of all the evidence and concluded that 'Swick's contribution shines through the dust of this scramble for priorities (1977)'.

At last in 1965, Swick was awarded the Valentine Award of the New York Academy of Medicine and he was introduced by the chairman (Melicow)—'And now 30 years have passed, 30 unkind years of heartache and oblivion'. At this meeting the great American urologists publicly apologized to Swick, followed by the award of many international honours and distinctions. But after a medical life-time of destructive criticism, and allegations of cheating and plagiarism, Swick was understandably upset, and when I (Grainger) traced and met him in New York in 1980, he was naturally still disturbed at the unfairness and unfounded criticism by his medical colleagues which had persisted over most of his professional lifetime.

In 1930, Uroselectan was superseded by two improved pyridone products both containing two atoms of iodine—Uroselectan B (Iodoxyl) [7.3] and Diodone, both synthesized by the Binz and Rath team.

The benzene ring was introduced in 1933 as a contrast agent by Swick and Wallingford (USA) but their molecule—sodium mono-iodo-hippurate—contained only one atom of iodine, was rather toxic and was not as satisfactory as Iodoxyl and Diodone.

In the early 1950's, Wallingford showed that the introduction of an acetyl-amino group in the meta- (C3) position of the benzene ring allowed the introduction of three atoms of iodine (C2,4,6 positions) and also greatly reduced the toxicity, increasing the LD50 by as much as ten times. Hoppe, Laren and others introduced a second acetyl-amino group at C5 and in the mid 1950's

the very much improved fully substituted tri-iodinated benzoic acid HOCM salts (diatrizoate [Urografin], iothalamate [Conray]) were introduced into clinical practice and became the standard contrast agents for more than the next 30 years.

The next major development occurred in 1969 when a young Swedish radiologist Torsten Almén [7.5], self-taught in organic chemistry, postulated that the high osmolality of HOCM salts was the cause of much of their clinical toxicity and that the osmolality could be reduced by transforming the molecule into a non-ionizing product such as an amide. Almén's original paper, entirely theoretical with virtually no chemical or clinical research, was understandably rejected by several major radiological journals but he eventually succeeded in publishing in *The Journal of Theoretical Biology* (1969)—a journal of which most radiologists were ignorant!!

Almén's ideas were then developed commercially and Metrizamide, the first triiodinated

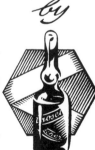
7.3 Advertisement for Uroselectan-B (*The British Journal of Radiology* 1933)

BRITISH CONTRAST MEDIA

in place of German preparations

PYELECTAN

BRAND OF IODOXYL INJECTION

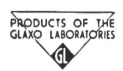

PRODUCTS OF THE
GLAXO LABORATORIES

Since its introduction on the Continent in 1931, this compound has retained its pre-eminence among contrast media for radiological

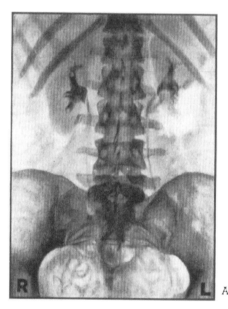

examination of the urinary tract. 'Pyelectan' is the name given to the Glaxo preparation of the compound. Reports have demonstrated that in density and definition of the shadow, in rate of excretion and in absence of reaction to the patient, 'Pyelectan' completely satisfies the highest standards. In pyelogram (A) exposed 3 minutes after injection of 'Pyelectan,' the pelvic shadows are already dense and clearly defined, the kidneys functioning well. The

right pelvis is seen to be slightly dilated and the diminution of the curve between the origin of the ureter and the lowest calyx

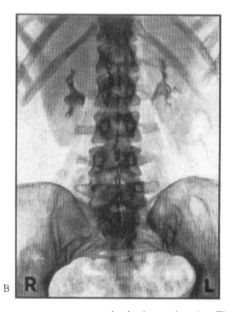

suggests a very early hydronephrosis. The ureters are shown more densely in the 3 min. pyelogram than in the 20 min. pyelogram (B); in the former they are slack and filled with solution; in the latter they are probably contracted. Exposure may be made 3 to 5 minutes after injection if kidney function is normal. In other cases the usual intervals are 10, 20, 30 and 50 minutes. For instrumental pyelography 'Pyelectan' (retrograde) is available.

PYELOSIL 'Pyelosil' brand of diodone injection unlike most other contrast agents, is non-irritant both by the intravenous and subcutaneous routes.

GLAXO LABORATORIES LTD., GREENFORD, MIDDLESEX. BYRon 3434

7.4 Advertisement for Pyelectan (Iodoxyl) (*The British Journal of Radiology* 1942)

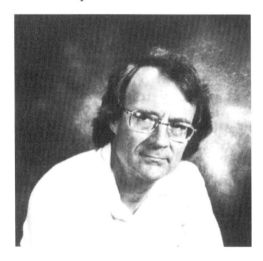

7.5 Torsten Almén

non-ionic low osmolality contrast media (LOCM) was marketed in the early 1970's, mainly as a myelographic agent for it was about 20–30 times more expensive than conventional high osmolality contrast media (HOCM) and too expensive for intravascular use.

Fortunately the pharmaceutical manufacturers soon greatly improved on the original Metrizamide and they synthesized and marketed the less toxic, more stable and much less expensive second generation LOCM. Iohexol (Omnipaque), iopamidol (Niopam) and ioxaglate (Hexabrix) were introduced in the mid 1980's and are still the contrast media of choice 10 years later.

Very recent developments have included the synthesis of the non-ionic dimers (iodixanol, iotrolan), each molecule of which contains 6 atoms of iodine and which are isotonic with body tissues at all concentrations. Although these products are more expensive than LOCM monomers, these non-ionic dimers may have some advantages for intrathecal and intravascular use.

During the 100 years since Röntgen's original discovery, the world of radiological contrast media has made enormous progress in clinical diagnosis, leading to unanticipated interventional diagnostic and therapeutic applications.

Despite the introduction of magnificent new imaging technology such as ultrasonography, CT and MRI, iodinated contrast medium research is still very active in improving the performance and reducing the toxicity of these essential imaging agents.

Our principal requirement at present is the production of contrast media of the same efficacy and low osmolality and toxicity of the second generation LOCM but requiring less expensive synthesis and capable of being marketed at lower cost to the consumer.

A well-illustrated account, with a bibliography, of the topics discussed above can be found in R.G. Grainger's 'Intravascular Radiology–the past, present and future' in the *British Journal of Radiology,* 1982, Volume 55.

8

British Military Radiology 1897–1919

'The discovery of the Röntgen rays and their use for the detection of hidden bullets has ... put a new weapon into the hands of the military surgeon.'

Though X-ray apparatus before 1900 was unable to penetrate thick parts, and produced images with poor definition, it could be used to detect fractures and metallic foreign bodies. Battlefield injuries could now be assessed prior to treatment. The Italians were the first to use X-ray diagnosis in war. The British followed, in 1897 using radiography in one of the Red Cross hospitals provided for the Graeco-Turkish war.

The difficulties of using X-rays in war became immediately apparent. Batteries and induction coils were heavy, an electrical supply was required for recharging, and battery acid was difficult to carry. The Crookes' tube and glass plates were extremely fragile. A dark room was needed for screening or developing radiographs. The whole process of radiography was time consuming, which caused stress when working under pressure. The surgeons in Greece concluded that X-rays would be very useful, but not at the front.

Surgeon-Major W C Beevor [8.1] faced these problems in 1897–8 in the Tirah campaign on the north-west frontier of India. He transported and used his X-ray apparatus in extreme cold and under primitive conditions. Ponies and indigenous troops with carrying poles were the only method of transport available.

The next military trial of X-rays was in the heat of the Sudan desert in September 1898, using the first two Army-issue sets. Wax insulation separating the wires of the induction coil threatened to melt. Run-down batteries were recharged by a dynamo driven by a pedal-cycle. (One of the cyclists later extolled the benefits of a motor-driven dynamo!) Despite the desert sand, Surgeon-Major Battersby obtained useful radiographs after the battle of Omdurman.

A year later war broke out in South Africa. 22,000 British soldiers were treated for wounds, injuries and accidents. Only a small proportion were examined using the nine army X-ray sets, as some were inoperative being incomplete or in hospitals without trained staff. The radiographer at the army hospital in Ladysmith continued to X-ray patients while under fire during the siege, recharging his batteries at a nearby mill. Voluntary organizations supplied much-needed auxiliary hospitals. At one, the Imperial Yeomanry

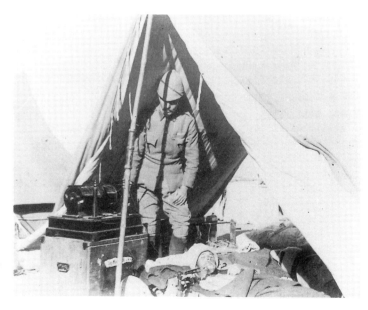

8.1 Surgeon-Major Beevor operating with the aid of X-ray apparatus on the North West frontier of India, 1897.

Hospital at Deelfontein, the pioneer Birmingham radiologist John Hall-Edwards produced high quality images in a room adjacent to the operating theatre.

In 1914 there were few full-time radiologists outside large cities, and none in the army. Although several radiologists were called up for service in the First World War, they found themselves performing unskilled tasks, while radiology was undertaken by untrained doctors, scientists and orderlies. Deployment improved during the course of the war. Skills developed in civilian practice were applied to chest, head and abdominal examinations. X-rays were used therapeutically for hyperthyroidism and to depilate skin used in plastic surgery. Foreign bodies were localized by stereoscopy or by a variation of the basic system devised by Sir James Mackenzie Davidson many years before. Electrotherapy was often practised by radiologists as an aid to rehabilitation.

More compact, powerful and efficient apparatus was available. General and base hospitals received radiographic sets early on. Casualty clearing stations were originally considered to be unsuitable for the type of surgery requiring radiological services, but with the onset of static trench warfare the role of surgery and radiology in these forward units increased. Bedside radiography became routine in hospitals which specialised in the treatment of fractured femur.

Without a mains supply, local electrical generation, usually petrol-powered, was essential. This was the outfit at the General Hospital at Rouen: one six inch Butts coil, a Zenith mercury gas interrupter, a wooden holder for the Macalaster-Wiggin gas tube and a table. Current was supplied by eight 1-in. square celluloid wet storage batteries and recharged by a one cylinder petrol engine. To assess severe wounds with sepsis and the likelihood of multiple foreign bodies the radiographers found that fluoroscopy (followed if time permitted by radiography) demanded an undercouch tube. Unfortunately this technique increased the radiation hazard from the poorly shielded X-ray tube.

The large numbers of wounded in the first weeks of the war required rapid improvization of temporary hospitals, at home and abroad, by the army and voluntary organizations. These often had neither radiology installations of their own nor provision of electricity. Mobile X-ray cars had been devised before the war to overcome this problem, but there were only two in the British army in January 1915. There was soon an *ad hoc* assembly of vehicles with dynamo, dark room and radiographic apparatus.

The London radiologist Archibald Reid and his army committee dealt with several technical matters including the design of mobile X-ray vehicles. Initially, the dynamo was powered by the vehicle's engine, but this produced unwanted vibration. Fourteen mobile X-ray units were sent abroad by the British Army: ten to France,

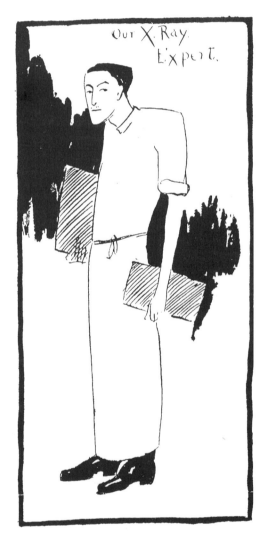

8.2 'Our X-Ray Expert'—a first world war radiographer in a military hospital in Birmingham during the First World War.

two to Salonika and two to Mesopotamia, many given by private donors. The British Red Cross provided several X-ray units for use in France and Italy. The Scottish Women's Hospitals had a mobile X-ray car in France [8.3] and another

industries the country relied on imports of gas tubes from America. The Coolidge tube was rarely available to the British army. By the end of the war arrangements for equipment design and testing, instructions on radiation protection,

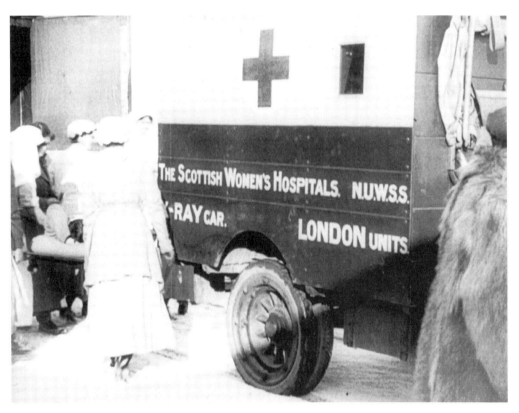

8.3 The X-ray ambulance attached to the Scottish Women's Hospital in France, 1917 (still from *The Scottish Women's Hospitals* in the Scottish Film Archive collection).

in Macedonia, as well as static apparatus in all their major hospitals. It proved more difficult to find skilled staff to operate them.

There was a shortage of X-ray tubes and electrical generators. Domestic X-ray manufacturers had suffered pre-war competition from Germany and there was a glass shortage. Britain did not produce the necessary soda glass, which had been imported from continental Europe. That supply had now ceased. Most of the instrument makers were called up for military service. Until government-directed research and manufacture achieved a revival of these

and training of orderlies in radiography and the care of equipment had been set up by the War office in Imperial College, London.

Wounded soldiers and sailors were transported back to Britain by ship. The army and navy had separate hospital transports and hospital ships. Many of the latter were equipped with X-ray apparatus. Naval hospitals and the larger battle ships possessed radiographic apparatus. The navy shared many of the problems of the army, with the additional trial of attempting radiography on a rolling deck.

9

Radiology in Paediatrics

One of the first X-rays taken in Britain, by Dr John Macintyre at Glasgow Royal Infirmary in 1896, was of the chest of a 6-months-old boy with a coin lodged in his oesophagus. Recognition of the potential of the new diagnostic method was prompt. Most children's hospitals had an X-ray machine within 15 years. The first radiologists were essentially technicians. Many years passed before their interpretative skills were acknowledged by referring physicians and surgeons.

Dr C. Teall, appointed to Birmingham Children's Hospital after the First World War, was among the first to train paediatric nurses to assist at X-ray examinations. Skill in talking to and handling a child, particularly an ill child, requires patience and training far beyond demonstrations of available immobilization devices—a truth still not universally admitted!

Knowledge of paediatric pathology is required by both radiographers and radiologists as much is unique to childhood, determining the examination required. Rickets and scurvy, common 100 years ago, have been superseded today by non-accidental injury and identification of obscure syndromes for genetic counselling, with malignant disease and problems associated with impaired immunity providing more work than straightforward infections.

While pioneers adapted apparatus to paediatric use and published some excellent work, such as Dr Teall's classical description of renal rickets, paediatric radiology was not recognized for more than 50 years as a speciality. Most radiologists spent too little time at children's hospitals to allow the acquisition of necessary background knowledge through regular contacts with clinical staff.

Not until 1948 was Dr Roy Astley appointed to Birmingham Children's Hospital as the first full-time British paediatric radiologist. His contributions have been many. *The Radiology of the Alimentary Tract in Infancy* was the first British radiology textbook confined to paediatric subject. In 1953 he acquired for 520 the first image intensifier for a children's hospital and commenced cinéangiocardiography. X-rays were produced by a GR electronic generator triggered by a simple switch on a Bolex 16 mm cinécamera and millisecond exposures were terminated with great accuracy. By 1968 an apparatus custom-built by Rank Medical allowed filming in 2 planes at variable angles. Cinéradiography was adopted to many other uses including the manometric study of the gastro-oesophageal junction in infancy by Carré and Astley in 1958.

In the 1970's remote controlled screening tables such as the CGR Pediatrix and the Siemens Infantoscope were produced specifically for paediatric use with cradles allowing X-ray examinations with minimal patient handling and loss of body heat. Diagnostic and therapeutic enemas in newborn and even in premature infants became safe techniques. The world market could not support such luxuries, although small cradles are still available for X-ray tables designed primarily for adults.

In the 1960s ultrasound revolutionized the work of most paediatric radiologists. Less expensive and, later, mobile apparatus producing non-ionizing radiation was a great advance. Ultrasound, although labour intensive, spread rapidly with encouragement from pioneers like Ian Donald in Glasgow.

In the 1990s magnetic resonance imaging though expensive is now established as a safe non-ionizing method which should be more widely available for children within the National Health Service.

Training in paediatric radiology was haphazard until The Royal College of Radiologists in 1980 accepted the recommendations of a Working Group chaired by Dr R.K. Levick of Sheffield, that, as more than 60% of X-ray examinations of children were controlled by radiologists devoting less than 50% of their time to paediatrics, all trainees should have a minimum of 3 months full-time training in a paediatric radiology department with further post-fellowship training available on request. In the 1990s superspecialization early in post-fellowship training in imaging modalities such as computed tomography, magnetic resonance, ultrasound, nuclear medicine and interventional radiology may leave radiologists responsible for examining children with only a minimum exposure to paediatric radiology and ignorant of basic paediatric pathology. The danger is a return to technician status if others can justifiably claim that they are better able to programme investigations.

The limited financial resources of the National Health Service and the increasing cost of advanced equipment leaves few children's hospitals able to offer every investigative modality on site. The increasing number of paediatric units within district general hospitals makes acceptance of designated paediatric radiologists and radiographers imperative to raise standards, reduce hazards and to veto unnecessary examinations.

In-service training sessions run by the British Paediatric Association Imaging and Radiology Group are open to all interested in paediatric radiology, whatever their commitment. The main forum for in-service training is the Annual Congress of the European Society of Paediatric Radiology, where British radiologists get to know one another and their colleagues from Europe, North America and the Antipodes. The first session in Paris in 1964 was attended by 14 British radiologists. Congresses have been held in London (1966, 1993), Birmingham (1973) and Glasgow (1985).

Since 1985 British paediatric radiologists have been involved in study groups of the World Health Organisation and the European Community/European Union producing guide-lines to improve the practice of radiology in paediatrics.

One Hundred Years of Radiotherapy in Britain

Introduction

Radiotherapy is defined as medical treatment using *ionizing radiation*, X- and gamma rays, alpha and beta particles, from X-ray and particle generators and from radium and artificial radio-nuclides. Over the last hundred years it has separated from the diagnostic uses of radiation and has become an independent specialty mainly devoted to treatment of cancer.

In the same way that diagnostic radiology has developed into *imaging*, using other methods as well as X-rays, therapeutic radiology has become *clinical oncology*, the study and treatment of cancer by chemotherapy and hormones as well as by radiation, in partnership with surgeons.

Two preliminary points should be made.

1 For many years much *non-malignant* disease was treated by radiation because:

(a) there *was* observed benefit;

(b) medical therapeutics was in its infancy; almost all effective drugs such as antibiotics, steroids and many others have only been introduced during the last 50 years.

2 Specialists in radiotherapy have continually needed much effort

(a) to become *independent*—separate from and taking over from dermatologists, surgeons, gynaecologists, and their colleagues the diagnostic radiologists;

(b) to obtain *full clinical control* and care of their own patients in their own hospital wards and clinics;

(c) to show that the consequent *benefits* of good specialized radiotherapy—cure in over half of all cancers and symptom relief for many of the others—*outweigh the hazards* of immediate tissue damage and long term carcinogenesis and leukaemogenesis.

These aims have now been almost universally achieved.

Radiotherapy has had an eventful hundred years, developing from an empirical footnote to diagnostic radiology, to become a major method of cancer treatment and a main component of oncology, side by side with surgery and medicine. Much of this has been developed in Britain. When we go back to treatment of disease in 1895 we need to be reminded that there were then few effective medical drugs, and that surgeons were limited by primitive anaesthesia and the absence of antibiotics to prevent or treat surgical infections.

The 1890s—speculation—empiricism—trial and error

Almost as soon as X-rays were discovered, biological effects were observed on the skin; this was not surprising since the rays then were virtually unfiltered and of very low energy and penetration. No one thought of any hazard, they were indeed described as 'invisible light' and were literally looked at. What we now describe as skin reactions were soon observed and were referred to as to as 'X-ray dermatitis'; epilation was also seen. The natural corollary was to use the 'light' to treat skin disease and this was the beginning of radiotherapy.

One of the first references to treatment (Lyon TH, Röntgen rays as a cure for disease, *Lancet* (1896) 1:326) suggested their use against bacteria, but the idea was soon given up.

Unshielded soft radiation from Crookes type tubes gave a disproportionately high dose to skin resulting in frequent heavy skin reactions and indeed 'burns' [10.1]. This was seen to cause epilation; one obvious deduction was that ringworm might benefit from X-ray treatment, and other skin diseases too; after all Finsen (ultraviolet) rays were already in routine use. Many hospitals already had 'Electrotherapeutic' Departments and these became the natural home for the new X-rays. Two of the earliest of these will be described.

At the London Hospital W.S. Hedley (1841–1930), already in charge of 'Electrotherapeutics' (first editor of the *Journal of Physical Electrotherapeutics* in 1900 and author of several books), took an early lead in using X-rays.

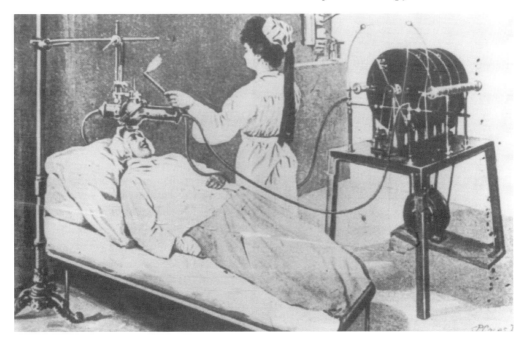

10.1 X-ray treatment in 1896–7: no screening or protection of patient or nurse.

Four of his pioneer 'X-ray operators' developed radiation injuries, dermatitis, and needed amputation of fingers or even hands—one of them, Ernest Wilson, died in 1911 from radiation induced cancer. Dr James Sequeira (1865–1948) a skin physician, treated rodent ulcers and ringworm. Dr Edward Morton (1865–1944) took over all treatment other than dermatological in 1903 and was succeeded by Dr Gilbert Scott, next Dr Geoffrey Boden, and then Dr Frank Ellis.

The Royal Infirmary, Glasgow, also developed radiology from the beginning. In 1885 Dr John Macintyre (1857–1928) was appointed 'Medical Electrician' in charge of an electrical room probably better equipped than Röntgen's own laboratory. Lord Kelvin (1824–1907) had been sent one of the first two copies of Röntgen's preliminary communication in January 1896 and this was passed on to Dr Macintyre. He may well have taken X-ray films as soon as or even earlier than Campbell Swinton had done in London. Large numbers of patients were soon referred, for treatment as well as for diagnosis. In 1901 over 1400 radiographs were taken. In 1902 a new electrical pavilion was opened including a Wimshurst machine built by Lord Blythswood. There were four rooms including one for diagnostic and therapeutic X-ray work, one of the first in the world under a medical specialist. Dr Macintyre gave a major address to the British Medical Association in 1914 on the use of X-rays and of radium in malignant disease. Dr James Riddell (1874–1935) became assistant in 1902, was the first whole time radiologist in Glasgow, and was appointed Lecturer by the University in 1916. His textbook was published in 1928. Sir George Beatson (1848–1933) began hormone treatment (by oophorectomy) and also used X-ray therapy in Glasgow after mastectomy for breast cancer from 1898; he was one of the first surgical oncologists.

Elsewhere in Britain

X-ray work of some kind began in 1896 or 1897 in most teaching hospitals in England, Scotland, Ireland and Wales. Centres in which much treatment was given in London included St Bartholomew's, Guy's, King's, Charing Cross, the Middlesex, the Cancer Hospital, and the West London Hammersmith Hospital. Notable work was similarly achieved in Belfast, Bristol, Dublin, Edinburgh, Leeds, Liverpool, Manchester, Newcastle, Southampton, and throughout the country.

Radiology was adopted by many physicians and surgeons as a new technical tool for both diagnosis and treatment, in the same way as was the microscope or stethoscope. Dermatologists, such as Sequeira at the London Hospital, were one of the first specialties to use X-ray therapy and they were to continue to have their own X-ray units for many years.

Much of the early treatment of cancer, other than for skin, was given by surgeons and gynaecologists using radium, to be discussed next.

1898 onwards—radium therapy

Within two or three years a second new, and apparently more effective, source of radiation became available. This was Radium, which had been discovered by Marie and Pierre Curie in 1898. Becquerel used to carry some in a pill box to demonstrate in his lectures, the box happened to be carried in a waistcoat pocket for a time. He soon observed the first human biological effect on his own skin, a typical blister—'moist desquamation'. Pierre Curie confirmed the finding and Becquerel himself consulted a dermatologist—Besnier—who noted the resemblance to an X-ray skin reaction and suggested there might be a similar therapeutic effect.

Radium, in needles or other containers, had the advantage that it could be inserted into body cavities such as the uterus, and even directly into tissue—interstitial radiation. Gynaecologists and surgeons became interested because the only effective treatment for cancer at this time was surgery, and many cancers were too advanced for the limited operations then possible. Surgeons such as George Beatson, Dawson Turner and John Macintyre were prominent in its use and the radiologists such as Robert Knox and Neville Finzi were equally interested, but suffered from the disadvantage of not being considered as clinicians to whom cases could come by direct referral from general practitioners.

The 1900s—over-enthusiasm for radium followed by reassessment and steady progress

Besnier's colleague, Danlos, began to use radium to treat lupus and other skin conditions with success, and published his findings in 1902. There was much early over-enthusiasm for regarding radium as a cure-all, which could be given to patients as a solution to be sipped or even injected! Many surgeons, not only British, but also Ewing at the Memorial Hospital in New

10.2 Patients having radium treatment for skin cancers in about 1900. They are holding applicators to their faces.

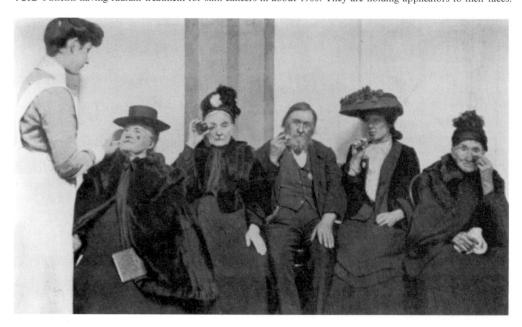

York, had regarded radium as no more than a caustic, to be given in a single massive treatment causing 'a slough in lieu of an excision' i.e. necrotic destruction. They were soon to be astonished by reading reports from Paris of cancers of the skin and tongue being cured without necrosis.

We must return to X-ray therapy. Assessment of the earliest years IS not easy now, nor can it have been easy at the time for the doctors concerned. Their X-ray tubes were unfiltered, there was no collimation, they were unreliable, inconsistent, and difficult to maintain.

A good contemporary source of information is the popular *Textbook of Radiology* written by Francis Williams, an academic Physician in Boston USA, with editions in 1901, 1902, and 1903. He read British, French, and German literature. His first edition omitted a full bibliography because it would have 'added nearly one hundred pages' and yet there was scarcely any reference to treatment. The second edition had forty extra pages, mostly on therapy, and in the third 'the therapeutic uses of the X-rays had grown rapidly in importance'. A list of about 250 therapy references was made up of about 80 general; 40 to X-ray dermatitis, injuries, and burns; 35 to cancer; 25 to lupus; 10 to rodent ulcer; 9 to bacterial infections; and about 15 to other skin diseases. Improvement is shown in illustrations of selected cases.

One important point at this early stage was the absence of any good method of measuring or expressing dosage, as stated by Williams: 'There is no wholly satisfactory way of measuring the intensity and quality of the light obtained by one physician with one apparatus as compared with that of another physician with different apparatus'. Williams gave good rules on 'length and frequency of sittings', suggesting treatment not more than twice a week 'to avoid X-ray dermatitis', continuing for up to six or eight treatments, repeating if there was recurrence and the skin was still satisfactory. He had also already developed simple collimation and shielding by enclosing the tube in a lead lined box, and using a mask with tin or lead applied to the face or skin.

When treating cancer it began to be realized that 'to produce a curative effect a so-called X-ray burn must be set up'.

Thus in summary benign diseases of the skin hypertrichosis and sycosis, ringworm, eczema and acne—could be treated by X-rays; but even at this early stage the most important disease to be treated was cancer, especially in the skin, but also in other accessible sites, such as the breast.

The 1910s—further development of radiotherapy comes from France

Work with Radium had continued. The Laboratoire Biologique du Radium was established in Paris by Wickham and Degrais, and Dominici became the father of deep radium therapy. Clinical work was developed further at the London Radium Institute from 1912, and at the Institut Curie from 1914. N.S. Finzi's book *Radium Therapeutics* appeared in 1913, and Dawson Turner's *Radium* in 1914.

We should now compare radium treatment with its predecessor X-ray therapy. Radium dosage was easier since one could begin to use milligramme-hours to express dosage almost from the beginning. The key book to quote was Wickham and Degrais' translated into English in 1910. It tells us how early containers such as rubber bags and ebonite boxes were soon discarded in favour of glass tubes or special applicators with either a metallic or linen base. Even a special uterine applicator was devised in 1908, mushroom shaped to cover the cervix with a stem to penetrate the uterine canal. With all these considerable benefit was derived for a few cases of cancers of the skin, breast, and cervix.

It is worthwhile quoting Dr Wickham's caution and integrity: 'I am not recommending radium as the ordinary treatment for breast cancer, I always advise that patients ought to be sent to a surgeon, and only use radium if the patient refuses surgery, or the surgeons consider the case inoperable'. Wickham usually considered X-ray therapy better for post-operative treatment because of its ability to cover a larger area. Many surgeons used radium at this time but continued to consider its use no more valuable or specific than any other caustic or cautery.

Progress during this decade and the next was being well expressed in British text books, especially Robert Knox's three editions of

Radiography and Radiotherapeutics published in 1915, 1917–18, and 1919, portraying well the general position before 1920. Dosage calculation was now becoming a routine. Knox advocated a combination of indirect measurement, recording time, voltage, milliamperes, distance from the source, and filtration; and direct measurement by the colour change in Sabouraud pastilles, or by the Kienbock measurement of blackening on strips of silver bromide paper enclosed in light-tight envelopes. The biological relationship to the erythema dose remained an additional practical check.

The choice of disease selected for treatment was beginning to be narrowed down. Considerable value was ascribed to the treatment of benign skin disease, skin carcinoma and rodent ulcer, other carcinomas and sarcomas, and leukaemia. Hodgkin's disease, often called lymphadenoma, was said to respond well, but it had not yet been appreciated that a 'disappearance dose' was insufficient to prevent recurrence. X-ray therapy was also recommended for treating 'benign hyperplasia' in various sites, exophthalmic goitre and uterine fibroma. Prophylactic treatment for post-operative cases of carcinoma was recommended.

Better X-ray tubes and better treatment were being derived from scientific development in continued partnership with diagnosis. Technical improvements continued in North America. In 1915 there was a great advance, the advent of the Coolidge hot cathode, high vacuum tubes producing 100–200 kV X-rays. This was followed by the gradual introduction of shock-proof generators and cables, and better shielding. Similarly cones and collimators began to be fitted on to the tube housing.

The 1920s—postwar improvement in radiotherapy

After the war British progress recommenced. The need for measurement of exposure or dosage was increasingly recognized, with consequent improvement and consistency in results of treatment. Tube development also advanced here as in America and 250 kV units appeared. It now became practicable to practise true '*deep X-ray therapy*' [10.3].

Treatment planning using multiple beams

began towards the end of this era. The hazards of normal tissue damage, and the need for protection began to be appreciated and investigated. The science of radiation biology began to be studied, though not yet under this name.

In 1919 there had been a dramatic finding in Paris. The results from radium implantation had been improved by Regaud and Coutard; they showed that by giving low intensity implants over 6 or 7 days using radium of 0.33 or 0.66 mg/cm activity, and similarly giving fractionated X-ray therapy over six weeks or longer, one could obtain complete skin and tissue healing after curative doses, a true landmark in this history.

Gynaecological treatment was similarly improved—the 'Paris system'. Later Forsell, Heyman and others developed one alternative—the 'Stockholm system' at the Radiumhemmet. These important changes were soon adopted in Britain.

Another landmark was achieved in 1928. Radiation dosage became steadily more precise, after the definition of 'R', the Röntgen unit, in 1928, with measurement and calibration by ionization chambers.

In 1929 (and as a second edition in 1940) Sir Stanford Cade published his *Treatment of Cancer by Radium*. This was almost the last major book on radiotherapy to be written by a surgeon, though many surgeons and gynaecologists were to continue to perform radium implants and insertions themselves for some time yet.

The 1930s—radiotherapy begins to become an independent specialty

The Radium Commission was established in 1929, to ensure that this very expensive material was used in medicine efficiently and competently. Radium centres were established and whole-time medical 'Radium Officers' were appointed; they naturally and sensibly also took over X-ray therapy, with generous co-operation from their diagnostic colleagues. In effect the specialty of radiotherapy had been founded. Whole time medical radiotherapists were thus beginning to be appointed from about 1930, for example at the London, University

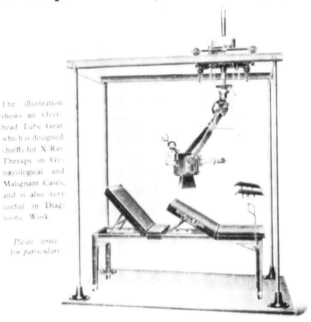

10.3 Accurate deep X-ray therapy apparatus used in the 1920s with full protection and beam direction from 200,000 X-rays.

College, and Royal Cancer Hospitals, and in Manchester, Edinburgh, Glasgow and elsewhere.

Another vital step had taken place earlier in 1919—the setting up of teaching and examination for the specialist Diploma in Medical Radiology and Electrology, the Cambridge DMRE, awarded from 1920 to 1942, the teaching coming under Dr A.E. Barclay for most of its later period. It had soon become the *sine qua non* for the appointment of any consultant radiologist; by 1942 over 500 had been awarded. The status of radiotherapy (and diagnostic radiology) was now recognized by the General Medical Council who decided in 1924 that teaching in radiology should be required from all medical schools. Diplomas were also awarded

by Liverpool in 1921, Edinburgh in 1926, and London in 1933, to become the main English Diploma in 1942 and to separate into DMRD (diagnosis) and DMRT (therapy).

The British Association of Radiologists was founded in 1934 and of Radiotherapists in 1935, soon combining and awarding their Fellowship by examination. The diplomas continued for some years as a required preliminary two years before the new Fellowship examination. The Association was to develop into a Faculty and thence to the present Royal College.

During the thirties there were substantial further improvements in radiotherapy equipment. In 1930 300–500 kV units became available and there were even the beginnings of megavoltage therapy. In 1931 Van de Graaff generators of 1-2 MV X-rays appeared, in 1934 Ernest Lawrence's Cyclotron and in 1935 the Metropolitan-Vickers million volt unit at St Bartholomew's. In 1934 the first primitive teleradium 'bombs' were constructed and in 1937 the Hammersmith Bryant-Symons 5g teleradium unit.

The 1940s—treatment becomes truly curative

During World-war II development again slowed, though some research continued with difficulties, until in 1945 the war ended with the dropping of atom bombs on Japan. Radiation carcinogenesis had by this time been observed, but was thought only to appear after high dosage tissue damage, it was soon to be seen in Japan in Hiroshima and Nagasaki, beginning with excess leukaemia occurring from 1947.

Key texts

Very important key texts were now published by two of the major figures in radiotherapy. In 1946 Sir David Smithers' *The X-ray Treatment of Accessible Cancer*, and in 1948 Professor Ralston Paterson's *The Treatment of Malignant Disease by Radiotherapy*. This latter Manchester book has gone through several more editions edited by successive Directors of Radiotherapy and is still current. Smithers and Paterson both began their books with the same premise, that curative radiotherapy could now be given for 'accessible cancers' (Smithers) or 'curable cancers' (Paterson)—of skin (including genitalia), mouth and lip, breast, uterus (cervix and body), and bladder. They also described the radiosensitive tumours (not yet necessarily curable) such as seminoma, medulloblastoma, and Hodgkin's disease.

Treatment principles

Principles of treatment were outlined for: tumour staging, choice of curative or palliative treatment policy, choice of technique, time and dose, multiple X-ray beam therapy and treatment planning, beam direction by moulds or shells, and finally radium dosage specification by

the Paterson-Parker Tables (1934 and 1938) for implants, 'mould' applications, and gynaecological insertions.

In 1946 the use of vitamin K was advocated by Joseph Mitchell of Cambridge as the first radiation sensitizer.

Wartime advances in nuclear physics led to the birth of another new specialty—nuclear medicine. In 1948 Artificial radioactive nuclides became available in the UK. Systemic treatments began, using iodine-131 for thyroid cancer and thyrotoxicosis, and phosphorus-32 for polycythaemia. Artificial radionuclides supplanted radium and radon for implants and insertions. Many different nuclides were used, dependent on their physical properties, especially isotopes of caesium and of iridium. Wires from the latter were of considerable value for implants as was well shown by Frank Ellis and many others. The major entry of the specialty into diagnosis and research also began.

The 1950s—a decade of change

There were four major changes at this time: the widespread adoption of megavoltage radiotherapy, the discovery and exploitation of the oxygen effect in radiobiology, the beginning of effective cancer chemotherapy, and the abandonment (with one notable exception) of radiotherapy for non-malignant disease.

Megavoltage radiotherapy

Megavoltage therapy, firstly from tele-cobalt units, and then from linear accelerators became the mainstay of external X- or gamma-ray therapy. It was accompanied by increasingly sophisticated simulators for planning.

The skin reaction ceased to be the main limiting factor for deep treatments. In 1951 the first *Tele-cobalt-60 unit* was constructed in Canada, spreading soon throughout Britain [10.4]. At almost the same time wartime advances in radar technology led to the development of the first clinical *linear accelerator* in 1952, the Hammersmith 8 MV unit with an isocentric head. This was rapidly followed by commercial production in 1953–4 of 4 MV linear accelerators to be installed in London, Manchester, Newcastle and elsewhere. It was ironic that

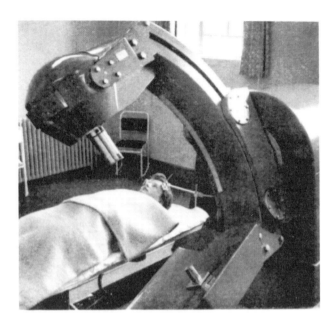

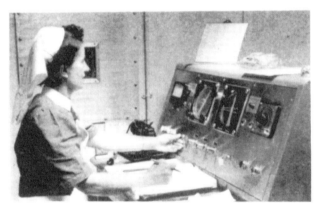

10.4 A radioactive cobalt treatment unit in the 1950s, delivering million-volt gamma-rays.

it was only just before this that in 1950 Dr Constance Wood's Medical Research Council Trial had shown no significant difference in biological effect between radium gamma-rays and 200 kV X-rays. The value of megavoltage radiation was of course derived from physical rather than biological reasons.

The oxygen effect

The oxygen effect was discovered by L.H. Gray in 1953, and its advantages were supported by Hugh Tomlinson in 1955, at the Hammersmith, leading to both successes and failures. The first new treatment to be derived was the use in 1955 of hyperbaric oxygen by Churchill-Davidson at St Thomas's, and the introduction of Medical Research Council trials of the method at Mount Vernon, Glasgow, and elsewhere. The method was never easy for patients, radiographers or doctors, and has been given up. Long term follow-up does show a small but significant advantage from its use, but it has been supplanted by hypoxic cell sensitizers, as will be seen below.

Cancer chemotherapy

In 1949 nitrogen mustard was used with astonishing effect for Hodgkin's disease and other lymphomas in London and Manchester. This was a remarkable discovery, coming from yet more wartime research work, on the effects of mustard gas. The death of radiotherapy was again foretold, to be supplanted by what became known as 'medical oncology'. Nevertheless it was to be many more years before other drugs were to follow and to be effective against other cancers, and today ionizing radiation continues to be used as much as ever.

Abandonment of radiotherapy

Immediately after the war many benign diseases were still being routinely treated, a few examples can be quoted. Ringworm remained common and contagious in children and it had been well treated by X-rays until effective antifungal drugs were introduced. It was shown much later that small numbers of skin cancers had been induced. Similarly ankylosing spondylitis, a painful crippling arthritis of British men, was very effectively suppressed by X-ray therapy, but leukaemia was found by Court-Brown and Doll to have occurred in 2% and radiotherapy has now been given up, after the advent of non-steroidal anti-inflammatory drugs. Low dose X-ray therapy was even being freely used for 'stimulation' of the pituitary gland and the ovaries for infertility. Earlier many other

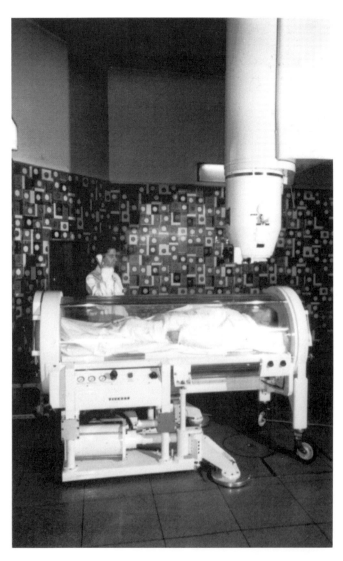

10.5 Treatment in a high pressure oxygen chamber by 4-million-volt X-rays in the 1960s.

diseases had been treated, apparently with benefit, such as asthma and tuberculosis, before effective alternatives became available.

The many long and productive studies of radiation carcinogenesis by Sir Richard Doll and others, the Reports from UNSCEAR (the United Nations Scientific Committee on the Effects of Atomic Radiation), and the studies of the Japanese atomic bomb survivors, have resulted in a public perception of the perils of ionizing radiation, probably now more than is deserved.

Thyrotoxicosis remains as the only common benign disease still treated by radiation, by X-rays in early times, now by radioiodine, without any carcinogenesis.

The first post-war books were followed by two important multi-author texts, to be used for many years: in 1955 Ernest Rock Carling. B.W. Windeyer and D.W. Smithers' *British Practice in Radiotherapy*, and in 1960 Ronald Raven's *Cancer*—a seven volume magnum opus.

The 1960s—consolidation and the introduction of computers and of automatic methods

Technology continued to burgeon during this decade, in two important ways. Manual insertion of radioactive sources had always been at least mildly hazardous and uncertain (though I am sure that Ralston Paterson would have denied this) and automated remote-control methods were introduced. In 1965 the Cathetron was brought into use at Charing Cross, as a method of remote controlled insertion of artificial nuclides in place of radium insertion, by O'Connell and Joslin. Computerized planning had by now come into use and the first international conference on the subject was held in Glasgow in 1967 under the inspiration of Charles Hope and Stuart Orr.

Two more attempts to exploit the oxygen effect were initiated. In 1966 Hammersmith Cyclotron neutron therapy began under Catterall and Bewley—following Jack Fowler's essential radiobiology in 1963. The treatment had to be given from a fixed horizontal beam, but the consequent practical problems were tenaciously overcome, and the initial results seemed highly promising. A second and better Cyclotron was installed in Edinburgh under William Duncan, a fully mobile isocentric head was available, and treatment became much easier. A different, more conventional treatment schedule was adopted, but the results were overshadowed by severe side effects. Limited treatment continues in Liverpool (and abroad), but the main medical uses of the Cyclotron are at present in proton therapy for eye tumours, and in production of positron emitters for scanning (PET).

In 1966 a new class of hypoxic cell sensitizers were introduced by G.E.D. Adams from Harwell. Trials continue without as yet a definitive answer.

The 1970s—the impact of effective chemotherapy and of modern oncology

The term 'oncology' (study and management of cancer) came into use at this time, and many more novel topics have been studied.

In 1970 combination chemotherapy began in the USA with MOPP (Mustine, Oncovin, Procarbazine, and Prednisolone—De Vita and others), for Hodgkin's disease, and combinations of drugs have become commonplace. From 1975 onwards there were many advances, such as the appearance in 1972 of bleomycin, the first drug effective against squamous cell cancers. Successful combinations have become effective against testicular tumours, particularly the radio-resistant teratomas. Bone marrow transplants have been widely used since about 1975, for leukaemia and very many cancers. Curative regimes have been found now for almost all tumours and leukaemias in childhood. 'Adjuvant' combinations such as CMF (Cyclophosphamide, Methotrexate, and Fluorouracil—Bonadonna 1977) have been introduced to add to other treatments in breast cancer. Modern hormone therapy has been developed for breast and prostate cancers, such as Tamoxifen and others.

Combinations of chemotherapy with radiotherapy have been devised for very many cancers. Trials of hyperthermia became common during this period, usually as an adjunct to X-ray therapy. This potentially promising addition to radiation has suffered from lack of knowledge of heat dose measurement, distribution and delivery, which are almost as primitive as was 19th century X-ray therapy.

The 1980s and '90s—technical improvements proliferate

The basics developed further; tumour localization has been undertaken by computerized tomography or magnetic resonance imaging; computerized treatment planning has become possible in three dimensions, with the aid of a simulator.

In 1986 continuous hyperfractionation (CHART) was begun by Stanley Dische and colleagues at Mount Vernon and significant benefit is now being demonstrated. Clinical trials became of greater value, using random controls and adequate statistical tests. Assessment of many trials together by meta-analysis has been developed by Peto and others. This has shown that persistent improvement in survival after adjuvant therapy of breast cancer is significant and long lasting. Integrated regimes have become common.

In 1982 the first edition was published of the text *Treatment of Cancer*, edited by Keith Halnan. A second edition came out in 1990 co-edited with Karol Sikora, and a third edition should appear in 1995.

Molecular biology

Molecular biology became a major force in the 1980s and 1990s. Knowledge of the structure, composition, and function of human genes, both normal and abnormal, including oncogenes, began to advance rapidly. Use of this information about cancer and many other diseases is leading to a new era in medicine. Today we are on the threshold of revolutionary new developments in prevention, diagnosis and treatment. Much work is being done, and there is great promise for the future. So far effective direct treatment is still on the horizon, but benefit has certainly been achieved from gene identification of tumour susceptibility in inherited cancers. One good example is medullary thyroid carcinoma in multiple endocrine neoplasia type 2, whose abnormal gene can now be identified with certainty at birth and its absence allows complete freedom from worry and need for regular screening. If the gene is present the child should undergo early thyroidectomy with certainty of cure.

Clinical results in practice

We should conclude with a look at the survival results that have been achieved, and approximate overall estimates are shown in Table 10.1. Radiotherapy and/or chemotherapy are used nowadays in about three out of four cancers, surgery continuing as a common first treatment but sometimes less radically.

These results come from combined treatment, and do not reflect the advantages of radiotherapy itself, as compared with surgery and chemotherapy. In general we should remember that surgery results in 100% removal of all the tumour cells in the tissue removed but is also mutilating. Chemotherapy at the other extreme treats the whole body, equally to all tissues, with the exception of those with limited blood circulation. Radiotherapy is limited to the

Table 10.1. Selected cancer survival rates.

	% survival at 5 years		
Site of cancer	1895	1945	1995
Basal and squamous skin	?10	90	100
'Head and neck'	?	40	80
Breast	?5	60	70
Uterus	0	65	75
Prostate	0	50	65
Bladder	0	30	50
Testis	0	40	80
Hodgkin's disease	0	30	80
Adult leukaemia	0	20	25
Childhood leukaemia	0	20	95
Overall	?5	30	55

volume selected, and has a selective effect upon the cancer cells within this, dependent on the tumour type and the radiation dose and time schedule. It is particularly valuable therefore in preserving important organs and functions such as the lips, mouth, the tongue and speech, the larynx and voice, the eye and sight, the breast itself even, let alone the hands, feet, limbs, and ideally normal body contours. Good quality of life is nowadays regarded nearly as important as life itself. Long term hazards are important for all treatments.

Conclusions

What have we achieved in this one hundred years? The survival results above show interestingly that at least as much has been achieved in the first 50 years as in the last, but we still fail to achieve improvement in the survival rate of patients with many of the common gastrointestinal and lung cancers, for which overall survival may be no more than 10–20%. It is fair to conclude that this first one hundred years has certainly witnessed substantial improvement but that the next should offer even more, and we or our successors still have much to do.

Radioactive Isotopes in Clinical Medicine and Research

The title for this historical review is the English version of Radioaktive Isotope in Klink und Forschung, the name for the stimulating International symposia held biennially in Bad Gastein since 1954 and organized by the 2nd Medical University Clinic of Vienna. The title accurately combines the two threads of the story: medical research with radioactive tracers and the establishment of procedures for clinical investigation (and, sometimes, therapy) which have, for the past 30 or so years, come to be classified as the province of 'nuclear medicine'. As Frederick Bonte remarked in 1979, referring to his experience in Cleveland, USA: 'Nuclear medicine began in a quiet way Just after World War II'. This account goes back to those beginnings—and to the previous 50 years—in a little detail and gives a broad view of the more recent developments.

1895–1945: the innocent years?

For nearly 40 years after Becquerel's discovery, in February 1896, of penetrating radiation from a uranium salt and Mme Curie's discovery in 1898 of the new element radium in uranium minerals, only the therapeutic applications of radioactivity established a secure role in medicine. However, among that peripatetic, cosmopolitan group of future Nobel prize winners who joined Rutherford for varying periods in Montreal, Manchester or Cambridge during those years was a 25-year-old chemist George de Hevesy who came from Budapest to Manchester in 1910 as a research student. At that time the concept of 'isotopes' was not firmly established. Challenged by Rutherford 'to separate RaD from all that lead' he failed, after 2 years' effort. But he joined Fritz Paneth in Vienna in 1912 and they worked together In chemical research, using RaD as an indicator for lead. He discovered the element Hafnium in 1923 and by 1934 had published 150 papers involving radioactive indicators in chemistry and biochemistry. He was awarded the Nobel prize for chemistry in 1943. When he died in 1966

nuclear medicine was just becoming accepted as a medical speciality.

Meanwhile, nuclear physics advanced steadily but for about 10 years, from 1928, came a series of inventions and discoveries that transformed the subject—and world politics. For medicine the critical event was the discovery by F. Joliot and I. Joliot Curie in 1934 that artificial radioactive isotopes are produced by irradiating certain elements with alpha particles and Fermi's demonstration three months later that they can also be produced by neutron bombardment of many different elements. Soon afterwards, in Copenhagen, Hevesy, with Chievitz (head surgeon of the Finsen Hospital) used a neutron source provided by Neils Bohr to prepare P32-labelled sodium phosphate for studies of phosphorus metabolism in rats. They published their results in *Nature* (November 1935) concluding that these 'strongly supported the view that the formation of bones is a dynamic process...'. This was the first study in the life sciences where an artificial radioactive isotope was used as an indicator.

From 1936 workers in the USA at Berkeley, Boston and New York used the isotopes Na24, P32, I128 and later I131 in biological and some clinical studies, with the cyclotron (Lawrence 1932) as source and Geiger-Müller tubes as detectors.

Limited possibilities for radioactive tracer work in humans now existed. But, in 1939, Meitner and Frisch, in Copenhagen correctly interpreted the outcome of neutron irradiation of uranium as nuclear fission. In Chicago, on 2 December 1942, Fermi operated the first self-sustaining chain-reacting pile. On 16 July 1945 Oppenheimer (who, in Robert Junck's 'beautiful years', 1923–1932, had taken his doctorate at Göttingen) supervised release of a genie of immense power for peace and war.

1945–1995: domesticating the nucleus

Within the UK two important political and administrative decisions combined with much enthusiasm and initiative in many hospitals and related institutions brought rapid progress in the use of the abundant supplies of new radioactive isotopes for clinical research which could lead to new diagnostic and therapeutic procedures. These were the decisions in autumn 1945, by the Government to set up the Atomic Energy Research Establishment, and by the MRC to set up an Advisory Committee on 'The Medical and Biological Applications of Nuclear Physics'.

From 1945 roughly every 10 years some particular event or development led to changes in direction or new opportunities as noted in what follows

1945–1955: Hiroshima to 'Atoms for Peace'

The US Government began releasing radioactive isotopes for specific projects in 1946. In Britain the research reactors GLEEP and BEPO were commissioned in 1947 and 1948 respectively and supplies of radioactive materials were soon made available, at modest cost. The National Health Service came into action in July 1948. The MRC Advisory Committee set up panels to approve applications for radioactive isotopes for medical projects, a system which remained in operation successfully for many years.

In Britain Ansell and Rotblat (Liverpool, 1948) were the first to use point by point counting to plot the distribution of I131 in patients. In the same year Norman Veall, at Hammersmith produced the important M6 counter for the assay of radioactivity in liquids.

In 1951 AERE and MRC co-sponsored a Radioisotope Techniques Conference in Oxford. 69 papers on medical and physiological applications were presented by speakers from 13 countries. In the opening paper Professor

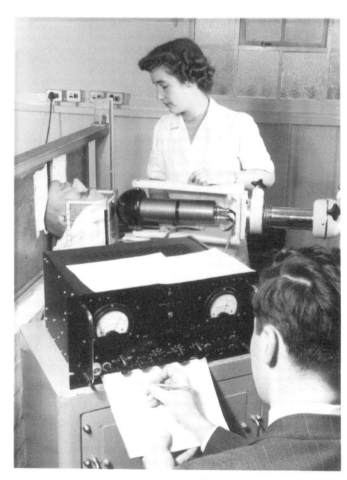

11.1 Manual scanning over a grid for brain tumours, using K42. Atkinson Morley's Hospital/Royal Marsden Hospital 1954.

Mayneord described his first automatic GM tube scanner; a month later Cassen (UCLA) published a report on his automatic rectilinear scaner, incorporating a calcium tungstate scintillation detector. At a second Conference, in 1954, Veall presented a new method of measuring cardiac output. His distinguished career in medical research with radioactivity lasted over 40 Years and took him to many countries.

The first Atoms for Peace Conference, sponsored by the United Nations, was held in Geneva in August 1955 and AERE supported a medical exhibit [11.2] to which several hospitals contributed material.

In addition, in 1955, the MRC Cyclotron Unit at Hammersmith was officially opened by Her Majesty the Queen. ·

A joint training programme was developed between a group of hospitals and an isotope school at Harwell. In addition, methods of preparing standards for the numerous new radioactive isotopes were submitted to inter-comparison between NPL, AERE, MRC Hammer-smith and the Royal Cancer Hospital over a number of years and a reference ionisation chamber developed, which is still widely used.

1955–1965: the advance of in-vivo techniques

Ten years in which backroom research moved into the clinic and the market, as Hal Anger in Berkeley perfected his gamma camera, the first commercially built scanners and later cameras appeared and whole body counters were developed for metabolic studies. But, as the number of photons needed to produce usable images raised problems in the radiation dose to the patient, research on imaging theory developed, with Professor Mallard in Aberdeen taking a prominent part then and for many years. In 1958, while still at Hammersmith Mallard built a

11.2 Part of UK Medical Exhibit, Atoms for Peace, Geneva 1955. The photograph shows clockwise: Mayneord's 3rd scanner; sample and *in vivo* measurements on Fe59; uptake of P32 in tumours of the eye; blood volume studies.

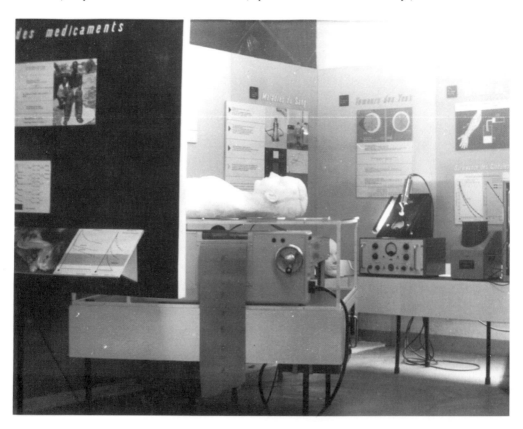

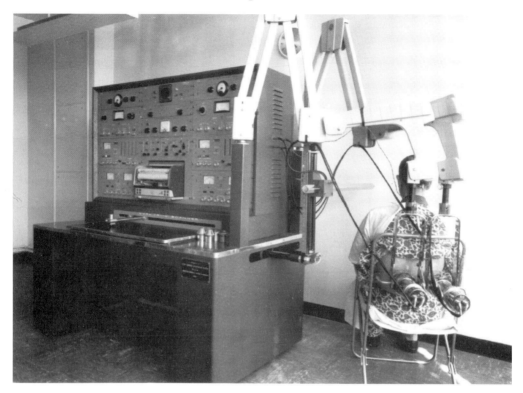

11.3 Tri D (multipurpose) scanner imported from California 1957. Photograph shows use for renography (Royal Marsden Hospital).

scanner used for brain tumour imaging and added a multicolour tape printer which provided a directly quantitative image. And then, in 1964, came Tc99m as the optimum choice of radioactive isotope for imaging with gamma cameras—work by Harper and colleagues from Brookhaven and Chicago which transformed the future of the subject, through the Mo99-Tc99m generator [11.4].

During these years a major programme for assessing the radiation dose to patients receiving radiopharmaceuticals was developed in the USA and the UK with great support from the US Society for Nuclear Medicine, founded in 1954.

A major outcome of the 1955 Geneva Conference was the formation of the International Atomic Energy Agency, in Vienna, in 1957. The Medical Division acquired a legendary reputation for organizing symposia and conferences which brought together medical radioactive isotope workers from all over the world, commencing in 1959 with the theme 'Medical Radioisotope Scanning'.

The British Nuclear Medicine Society was founded in 1965 and similar bodies were being created all over the world. Similarly, academic and practical training in nuclear medicine advanced, with, in Britain, the formation of the Institute of Nuclear Medicine at Middlesex Hospital Medical School in 1961 and the introduction of the MSc in Nuclear Medicine in London University in 1970.

1965–1995: chips, computers, cyclotrons, tomography

In 1964 Kuhl and Edwards (Philadelphia) produced their transverse axial emission tomography system. Thermionic valves began to disappear with the advance of the transistor, the printed circuit and the chip. Small powerful digital computers appeared. Hofstadter's alkali halide scintillator of 1948 had triumphed. And in 1972 came X-ray CT.

There followed 20 years of adjustment as the new technology was incorporated into nuclear medicine and the possibilities began to be

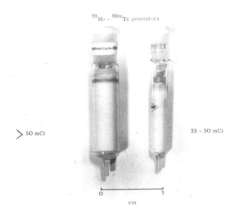

^{99}Mo - ^{99m}Tc generators

> 50 mCi   25 - 50 mCi

0   5
cm

11.4 Mo99-Tc99m generators *c.* 1968:
half life Mo99: 67 hours;
half life Tc99m: 6 hours;
(single photon 0.14 MeV).

explored. At Hammersmith, in 1980, the MRC Cyclotron Unit celebrated its Silver Jubilee: a remarkable record, with 60 different radioactive isotopes investigated and 56 radiopharmaceuticals created for just 6 isotopes. In 1967 they produced their prototype Rb81-Kr81m generator: by 1980 they were distributing 30 generators per week to UK hospitals. It has been estimated that in the year 1989/90 16,400 lung scans using this generator were performed in the UK. In 1979 a positron emission tomographic (PET) system was installed; in 1987 the original cyclotron was replaced with a commercial instrument which produces 40 MeV protons and their long programme of physiological research should now continue for many years given adequate support.

Elsewhere a variety of single photon CT systems have been studied—some home built, especially in Aberdeen, others commercial models, all with the background of new radiopharmaceuticals and efforts to use monoclonal antibodies. Other hospitals have begun to acquire their own cyclotrons. And some 10 years collaboration between the Rutherford-Appleton Laboratory and the Institute of Cancer Research, with cyclotron support from Hammersmith and Birmingham has led to a successful multiwire proportional counter positron emission CT system.

Altogether, a remarkable story of a century of world wide collaboration between workers in all branches of science, medicine and engineering.

The Invention of Classical Tomography and Computed Tomography (CT)

Tomography means 'slice imaging'. A conventional planar X-radiograph is a 2D image of a 3D structure and hence contains no depth information. It is a projection image in which the X-ray intensity arriving at a point in the image is a function of the X-ray absorption along the straight line joining that point to the source, as well as a function of off-line structures due to scattered radiation.

A (classical) tomographic image is formed when the source and the detector move in some coupled way so that each ray joining the source to each detector point pivots about a point in an 'in-focus' plane. The pivots for all the rays joining the source to each detector point all lie in the same plane. Rays still pass through other planes but the structures in these out-of-focus planes is simply blurred by the movement and smeared across the in-focus plane. By adjusting the pivoting, different planes can be brought into focus. The movement can be linear, circular or spiral; in fact anything satisfying the above constraints. Each has merits and disadvantages. Conventional planar radiographs can be difficult to interpret because of overlying structures.

Who invented classical tomography was hotly disputed in the 1930s and 1940s. Many scientists were independently working entirely in ignorance of each other in different countries. The details of how they found out about each other's work and what happened then is a fascinating story which I have told elsewhere (Webb 1990).

If these workers are listed chronologically, then the French dermatologist André Marie Edmond Bocage invented tomography, patenting the technique on 3 June 1921. However he was not involved in constructing equipment until the late 1930s. On the other hand the Dutch radiologist, Bernard Zeidses des Plantes [12.1] built equipment in 1922 but did not publish until a series of papers starting in 1931 and a seminal doctoral thesis in 1934. His apparatus formed the basis of the first commercial equipment by Massiot. The Italian Alessandro Vallebona, the Germans Ernst Pohl and

Gustave Grossmann, the French Felix Portes and Maurice Chausse and another Dutch-Canadian Bartelink also independently invented classical tomography between 1921 and 1934. Around 1934 they began to find out about each other and the literature contains some steamy rows. Tomography was a hot topic and the stakes were high. Diagnostic radiology was being revolutionized. Zeidses des Plantes is widely credited with the pioneering developments. Born in 1902, he was scientifically active until his death in 1993 and was able and willing to provide a retrospective on the early events of the century in a series of letters to me in 1988.

After 1934 a number of clearly derivative workers constructed tomographic apparatus. Jean Kieffer and Robert Andrews independently brought the method to America. Edward Twining constructed apparatus in the UK and the British radiographer William Watson began a

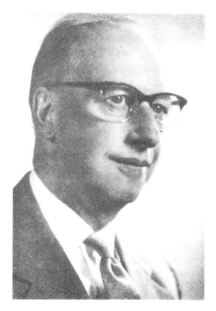

12.1 The pioneer of classical tomography, Professor Bernard Zeidses des Plantes (from Bruwer (1964) *Classic Descriptions in Diagnostic Radiology* Vol 2. Courtesy of Charles C Thomas, Publisher, Springfield, Illinois).

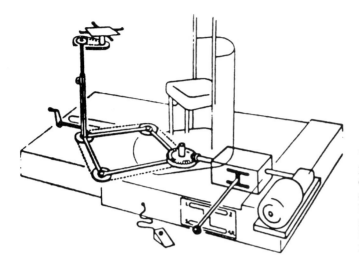

12.2 The method of corotating the patient and detector in the Mark 2 equipment of Watson for transverse axial tomography (the Sectograph). Note the use of the Austin 7 gearbox to vary the speed (from Stephenson (1950) *Brit. J. Radiol.* **23**, 319–334).

long career in developing ever better methods of section imaging. His invention with patient and film corotating in a glancing fan of radiation was in use well into the 1960s [12.2].

A 'computed tomography' image (or CT slice) is a true section. It is the X-ray picture of a slice of the patient which would be formed if a real slice of tissue could be extracted and a radiograph taken of it. Of course the technique is in reality non-invasive. A CT image is unblurred by adjoining sections. An X-ray source and detectors move relative to the patient and take thousands of projection images from which CT sections are reconstructed by mathematical techniques. The final black and white image is an analog reconstruction of the digital information and can be manipulated and interrogated on a television display. In the early machines both scanning and reconstruction took many minutes but now sub-second CT scanning is common with virtually real-time image generation.

Who invented CT? Again there is no simple answer. The practical invention is rightly credited to two scientists Allan Cormack and Godfrey Hounsfield who shared a 1979 Nobel Prize for the invention. Cormack had worked on the maths and early experiments as long ago as 1956. Hounsfield and EMI created a practical scanner [12.3].

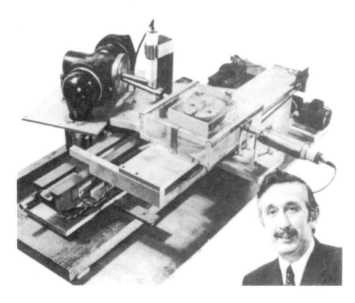

12.3 Sir Godfrey Hounsfield and the laboratory prototype equipment for CT (From Oldendorf (1980) *The Quest for an Image of Brain: computerized tomography in the perspective of past and future imaging methods*, Raven Press, New York.

Announced at the 1972 BIR Congress, work had started in 1967 and within a few years after 1972 there were hundreds of CT scanners throughout the world. It was the greatest quantum leap in radiology since Röntgen's discovery. The combination of the industrial talents of EMI, clinicians at London's Atkinson Morley's Hospital and the investment of the UK Department of Health got the EMI-scanner off to a good start.

Rooting around the literature however one can find many who might have invented CT. The

reputedly built in Kiev in 1957 for medical purposes. William Oldendorf in the US had grasped the principles. Similar ideas underpinned David Kuhl and Roy Edwards' apparatus for emission CT (radioisotope section imaging) in the 1960s and they had a primitive transmission CT scanner in 1965 [12.4]. None of this retrospective should detract from the practical achievement of routine clinical X-ray CT in 1972; all these earlier developments must be viewed with the wisdom of hindsight.

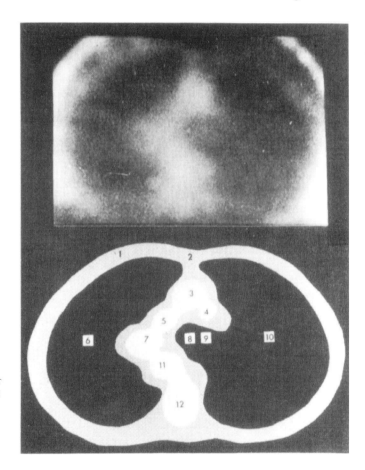

12.4 Possibly the world's first CT scan of a patient on 14 May 1965 made with a modified Mark 2 emission CT scanner by Kuhl and Edwards (courtesy of Dr David Kuhl).

mathematics of reconstruction from projections goes back at least to Radon in 1917. Gabriel Frank patented most of the method in 1940. Shinji Takahashi reinvented many of the steps in Japan throughout the 1940s. A CT scanner was

Classical tomography has virtually disappeared. CT is now so common, the miracle is almost taken for granted. Despite contemporary developments in MRI, the unique role of CT is here to stay.

Nuclear Magnetic Resonance

The phenomenon of magnetism has been recognized since the 6th century BC but the first reference to a magnetic instrument is by Wang Chhung, a Chinese sceptic who described a south pointing ladle in 83AD. The ladle, the shape of which was based on the great bear constellation, represents the ancestor of all dials and pointers—indeed the oldest instrument of all magnetic and electrical science. The first account of a magnet in the West is in a letter from a French military engineer, Pierre de Maricourt better known as Peter Peregrinus.

This letter, one of the first European scientific documents of the Middle Ages, gives a detailed description of the compass. It was not until 1600 however, that William Gilbert, Queen Elizabeth I's physician, in his monumental work *De Magnete* set out the scientific evidence for the earth itself behaving like a giant magnet. Gilbert invented the phrase 'terrestrial magnetism' and the word 'electricity'.

In 1820 Oersted in Copenhagen observed that an electric current could produce a magnetic field and in 1831 Michael Faraday at The Royal

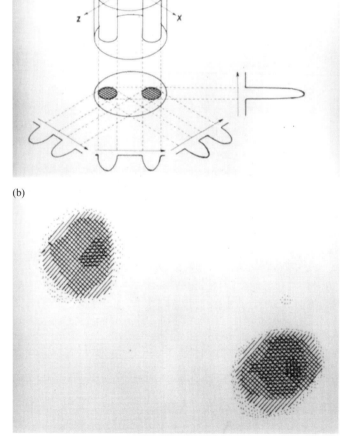

(a)

(b)

13.1 The first MR image: transverse sections of two tubes of water (Lauterbur 1973).

Institution in London described the phenomenon of electromagnetic induction. James Clerk Maxwell took the unifying lines of force invented by Faraday and in 1865 brought the separate topics of electricity and magnetism together in four simple formulae—Maxwell's equations. His electromagnetic theory of light was one of the great unifying statements of physics.

The fact that certain atomic nuclei might behave like small bar magnets by virtue of their spin and associated electrical charge was postulated by Pauli in 1924 and the possibility of a resonance method for detecting such nuclear magnetic moments discussed by several workers in the 1930's. Rabi of Columbia University demonstrated the phenomenon in a molecular beam in 1939 but it required the stimulus of the Second World War to provide the appropriate electronic techniques to enable the first demonstration of nuclear magnetic resonance (NMR) in matter to be achieved. Felix Bloch in Stamford and Edward Purcell in Harvard building on Rabi's work placed atoms with an odd number of particles in their nuclei in a strong magnetic field and then perturbed their orientation with a brief pulse of radio frequency radiation. Atoms of appropriate resonant frequency responded with a minute radio frequency signal which could be measured. The results of these experiments were announced almost simultaneously in 1946. Bloch and Purcell later shared the Nobel prize for their discovery.

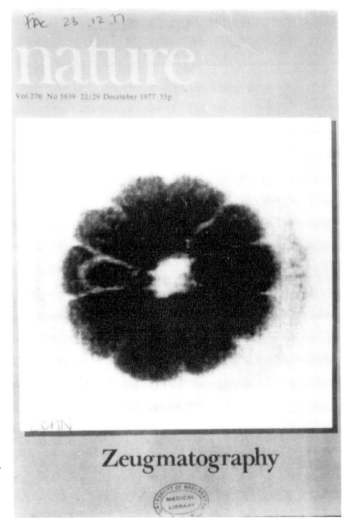

13.2 Transverse sectional image of a lime (Andrew et al 1977). The term Zeugmatography was devised by Lauterbur.

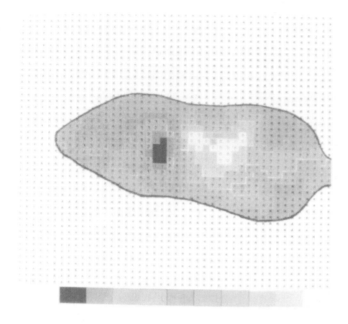

13.3 Mouse image (Mallard 1974).

Over the next few years NMR was detected in all forms of matter. The phenomenon became an important tool for the study of matter at the molecular level and has widespread applications in engineering, archeology and space research.

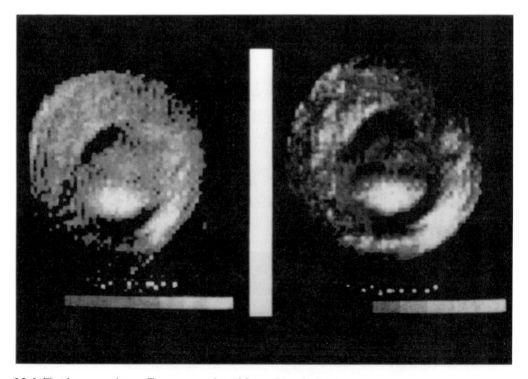

13.4 First human MR image. Transverse section of finger (Mansfield and Maudsley 1976).

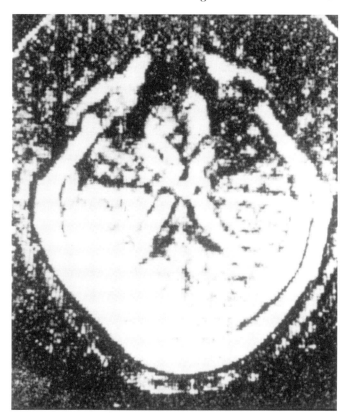

13.5 Transverse section of head
(Clow and Young 1978).

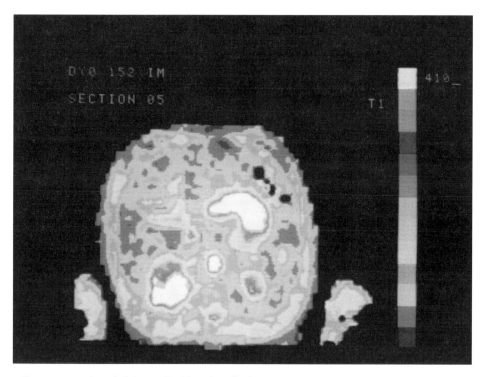

13.6 Transverse section of abdomen (Smith and Mallard 1980).

(a)

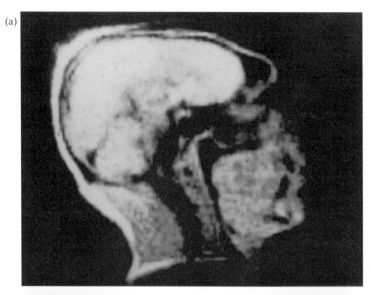

(b)

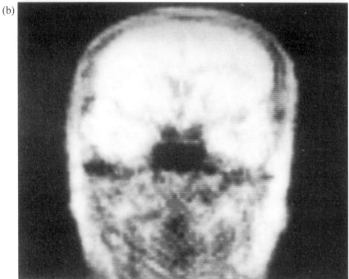

13.7 Coronal and sagittal sections of the head (Holland et al 1980).

The earliest biological experiments on living subjects with NMR were conducted by Bloch and Purcell in 1948 but it was not until advances were achieved in magnet technology in the 1960's that high resolution NMR spectra in one and two dimensions became possible. Since NMR spectral lines are very close together it was necessary to develop magnets with very uniform fields. During the 1970's high resolution NMR spectroscopy was applied to living tissue with recordings of ^{31}P, ^{1}H and ^{13}C.

In 1973 Mansfield and Grannell in Nottingham described NMR diffraction in solids. Multiple pulse line narrowing sequences and a magnetic field gradient provided spatial resolution. In the same year Lauterbur in a letter to *Nature* demonstrated a 2D image of two tubes of water [13.1] arguing that if a gradient field was applied to a structured object each nucleus would respond with its own frequency determined by its position. Reconstruction of the object could then be carried out by the type of computer algorithms being proposed for X-ray computed tomography. The conjunction of magnetic and radio frequency fields led him to coin the word *zeugmatography* (Greek for 'joined together').

An MR image is a 2D representation of the NMR signal from resonant nuclei in a thin slice. The sensitive point and line scanning methods introduced by Hinshaw in 1974 were important but have now been superseded by planar imaging. Definition of a slice is usually achieved by a selective excitation method first described by Garroway and others in 1974 and unusually implemented by the spin warp technique of Edelstein and Hutchison *et al* described in 1980. From 1974 to 1978 a variety of images were produced of fruit [13.2], vegetables and animals [13.3].

Damadian had suggested in 1972 that NMR might be exploited in the diagnosis of human disease. The first live human NMR image to be reported was a cross-sectional proton image of a finger by Mansfield and Maudsley in the *British Journal of Radiology* [13.4]. (Proton ^{1}H is the most abundant nucleus in the body, present in both water and fat. It also has the highest magnetic moment.) Demonstration of the potential of the technique with small bore systems was followed by the non-trivial task of scaling these systems up to whole body size. The first human whole body MR image was of the thorax by Damadian in 1977. Others quickly followed with transverse sections of the head [13.5] by Clow and Young at the Hammersmith hospital, the abdomen by Mansfield and others in Nottingham and the abdomen [13.6] and thorax by Smith and Mallard in Aberdeen. In 1980 coronal and sagittal images of the head [13.7] were published by Holland *et al* from

Nottingham together with the first images of intracranial pathology [13.8] by Hawkes, Holland Moore and Worthington. The difficulty in separating tumour from surrounding oedema subsequently provided a stimulus to develop contrast agents based on paramagnetic moieties.

An essential requirement of human MR imaging is a magnet with a bore of sufficient size to accommodate the whole human body and capable of generating a uniform field. Early whole body scanners were air core resistive solenoids producing magnetic fields up to 0.15 tesla and restricted to transverse images. To achieve higher field strengths superconducting solenoids are now generally used. Oxford Instruments in the UK were pioneers in the development of superconducting magnets which opened up clinical imaging. The first such system for clinical use was in the Hammersmith Hospital in 1981. By 1983 the first commercial MR scanners were being installed with an increasing number of cryogenic systems generating higher fields up to 2 tesla over the next decade. Multi-slice techniques provided a more efficient use of time; MR images can now be obtained in fractions of a second—approaching real time using an echo planar technique first proposed by Mansfield in 1977.

Although the phenomenology underlying tissue contrast in magnetic resonance imaging remains incompletely understood, a substantial data base of the signal characteristics in human pathology has been built up as its multi dimensional facility has been explored.

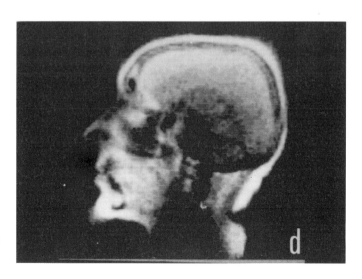

13.8 First MR demonstration of intracranial pathology (Hawkes, Holland, Moore and Worthington 1980).

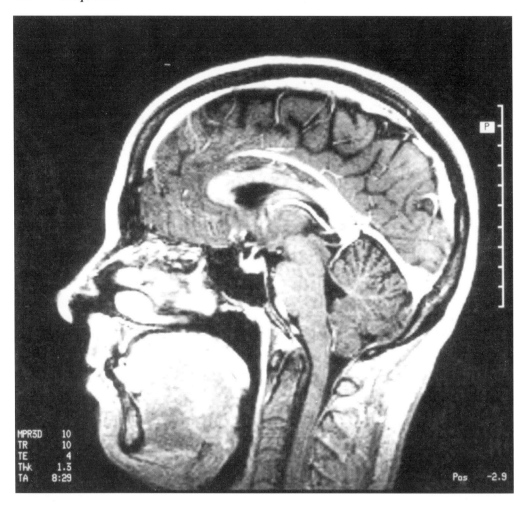

13.9 Modern MR sagittal section of the head depicting detailed anatomy of the brain.

MR imaging is now an accepted and widely used diagnostic modality for clinical radiology specially in the evaluation of pathology in the nervous system [13.9], the musculo skeletal and the vascular systems. Functional, interventional, spectroscopic and microscopic MR imaging are all currently under development for clinical use in this fast expanding field.

'Inaudible Sound'—Medical Ultrasound

It is estimated that ultrasound now accounts for forty per cent of all medical diagnostic imaging and that there may be as many as 100 000 machines in the world. As the first successful steps were taken in the 1950s this represents an astonishing rate of growth. This very short chapter cannot do justice to the immense amount of work by innumerable people that made this possible; it can only give a simplified view and mention the work of a few individuals.

The foundations of ultrasound were laid by the Curies, Paul Langevain (1872–1946) and the pioneers of echo sounding and submarine location in the 1910s and 20s. The loss of the *Titanic* and submarine warfare stimulated research on underwater acoustics. Then the Second World War brought advances in electronics and by the late 1940s ultrasound was being applied to the detection of flaws in metal components. A-Scan instruments were developed by Firestone at the Sperry Corporation, in Japan by Ichida and in Scotland by Sproule at Kelvin & Hughes. By 1948 the medical potential had been recognized. From this point advances were dominated by a few individuals and small groups: in Glasgow, Donald, MacVicar and Brown (obstetrics and gynaecology); in Denver, Holmes and Howry (general medicine); and in Sweden, Edler and Hertz (cardiology). The use of Doppler ultrasound for fluid flow measurement can be traced back to the 1940s. A decade later Satomura in Japan was measuring blood flow.

Ian Donald and his colleagues made significant contributions to the medical use of ultrasound, Donald's attention was drawn to the medical possibilities of ultrasound during a lecture in London by J.J. Wild from Minneapolis. After moving to Glasgow one of Ian Donald's patients put him in touch with the heavy engineering firm of Babcock & Wilcox and experiments ensued with the companies' 'supersonic' flaw detector. Next came cooperation with Tom Brown of Kelvin & Hughes and this resulted in the development of the first contact scanner [14.1]. The transducer on this machine moved freely in one plane while being kept in contact with the patient thus avoiding

the water bath favoured by other experimenters. Brown saw this not only as a natural development from industrial practice but also as necessary to work with the sick elderly patients in Donald's gynaecology wards; Brown described the first images as 'rather disappointing' [14.2] After years of experiment in an atmosphere of scepticism small numbers of static scanners were produced; these were the Diasonograph (Kelvin & Hughes, Smiths and later Nuclear Enterprises) and the Porta-Scan (Physionics/Picker). These slow cumbersome machines established the place of ultrasound and showed its possibilities in obstetrics and gynaecology, general medicine, cardiology and ophthalmology. All these were explored and clinical techniques were developed and tested.

Then in the early '70s the real-time revolution started. At first the images had few lines, poor resolution and a limited field of view and were aimed at visualizing moving structures. Only gradually was it realized that real-time could be of value on any part of the body. The advantages are now clear; easy to use and learn to use, the machines are smaller and easier to demonstrate and install. These advantages led to wider acceptance, increasing sales and increasing investment in research and development.

Looking back it can be recognized that 'real-time' started in 1950s with Wild's transducer oscillating at a few sweeps per second while scanning in a water bath around a patient's neck. The first array appeared about 1965; this was a 10 element concave transducer built by East German ophthalmologist, Werner Buschmann and Kretztechnic of Austria. Of much greater impact at the time was the Vidoson that appeared in 1967. This remarkably simple machine designed by Richard Soldner of Siemens used a transducer rotating at the focus of a parabolic mirror in a water filled enclosure. This was overtaken by a return to the array principle. Bom developed small arrays specifically for cardiology. In 1974 the first commercial linear array scanner appeared; this was the ADR2130 from Advanced Diagnostic Research in Arizona. Development became intense so for example by 1979 eleven forms of real-time

(a)

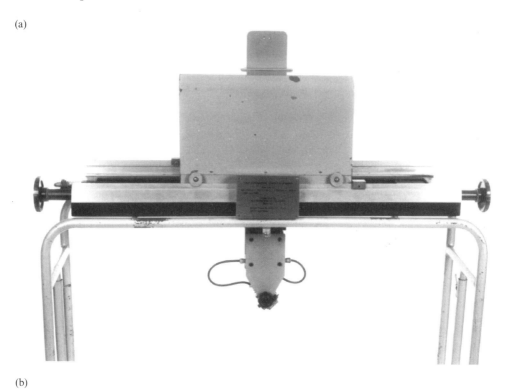

(b)

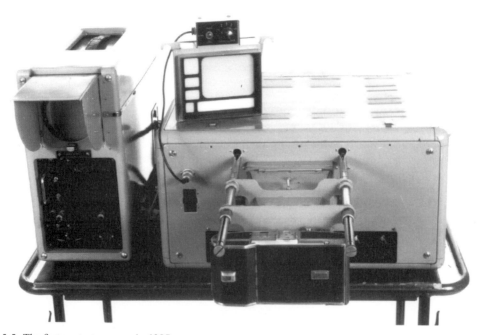

14.1 The first contact scanner (*c.* 1956).
(a) The scanning mechanism built on a hospital bedtable. Transducer 1.5 MHz.
(b) The electronics; a Kelvin & Hughes Mk 4 Flaw Detector(left) and the section-scan display unit (right) with Polaroid camera to record the scan which took a few minutes to perform. The data recording unit (connected by cable) allowed hand-written information to be photographed onto the scan picture.

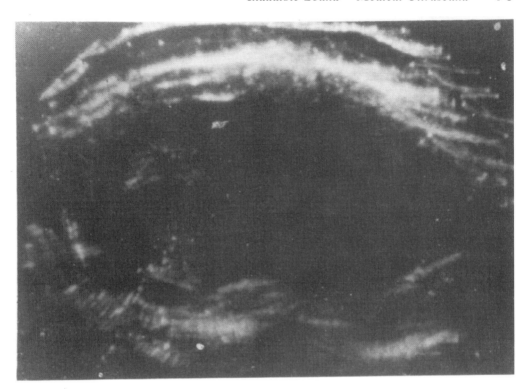

14.2 An early image from machine in [14.1]. This shows a pregnancy at 14 weeks, echoes from fetus towards left. Provisional diagnosis was fibroid.

transducer were described. In parallel, Doppler progressed from simple fetal heart detectors and blood velocity meters to pulsed systems able to measure flow at selected depths. Then pulsed Doppler was combined with real-time to give duplex scanners. From these have grown systems giving a dramatic display of flow in colour superimposed on high resolution cross-sectional images.

From the very beginning 3D has been a goal; now with the power of microprocessors this has become a reality for specialized use. It is tempting to see such achievements as the ultimate but it is more likely that with the continuing co-operation of medics and paramedics, physicists, engineers and industrialists, ultrasound imaging will continue

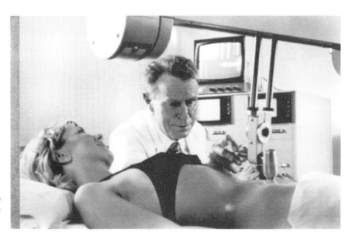

14.3 Professor Ian Donald using a Nuclear Enterprises NE 4201 static scanner, about 1977.

to develop and applications advance as rapidly as ever.

*

The history of medical ultrasound is being recorded by the British Medical Ultrasound Society which is developing a historical collection with the assistance of the University of Glasgow. A similar relationship exists in the USA between the American Institute for Ultrasound in Medicine and the National Museum of Medicine. Both collections are keen to receive offers of material of all kinds relating to the history of ultrasound.

15

Radiation Dosimetry

Soon after the discovery of X-rays by Röntgen in 1895, and of radioactivity by Becquerel in 1896, electroscopes and electrometers were utilized to study the emitted radiations. However, they were not employed for the measurement of dosage until 1905 when Franklin realized their possible advantage over pastille and photographic methods already in use.

The need for quantifying dosage had become apparent from the biological effects of the radiations, namely erythema, epilation and necrosis, and pastille and photographic techniques were initiated in 1902. Holzknecht produced a pastille radiometer based on colour changes of certain chemicals when irradiated, but his system did not prove satisfactory. The first practical method was developed by Sabouraud and Noiré in 1904, and such techniques remained in use until the 1930s [15.1].

Photographic radiometers were first used by Stern, also in 1902, and Keinbock produced his quantimeter in 1904, though this approach had limitations. In later years, this method proved reliable in distribution measurements and for protection-level monitoring.

Returning to the ionization approach, after Franklin had produced his special electroscope in 1905, others developed the technique further [15.2], including Villard [1908], and Szilard [1914] who set down detailed requirements for a practical instrument. During the next few years, a number of authors considered the question of a unit of dosage, which will be considered below. Indeed, ionization was to become the method of choice for precision measurements and standards.

15.1 Pastille radiometer. Irradiated pastille (upper half circle) colour-matched to one of 24 shades (lower half circle) on rotatable disc.

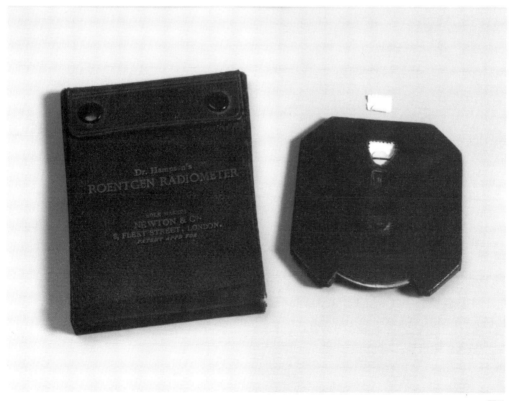

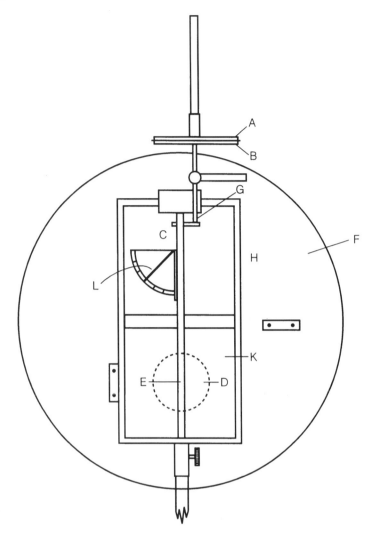

15.2 Modified Franklin electroscope. Gold leaf L in upper chamber. Air gap E irradiated through set aperture D in lower chamber (1906).

First, mention must be made of other approaches to the measurement of dosage, including fluorescence techniques (1907), the change in the resistance of selenium when irradiated (1915), and the development of formulae for the calculation of relative doses based on the physical parameters concerned in the irradiation. By 1920, various 'erythema doses' were postulated, making direct use of the biological response, but all these approaches had inherent limitation.

In parallel with the evolution of the measurement of the quantity of radiation, the specification of its quality also received attention. Röntgen

himself had demonstrated the variation in penetrative power of X-rays, and as early as 1902, a step-wedge penetrameter was used to distinguished between 'hard' or 'soft' radiation. Concepts of half-value layer (1912), absorption coefficient (1914), peak kV (1918) and effective wavelength (1922) were introduced as specifications.

Returning to the development of units of measurement, this initially concerned the work of individuals, but later became a matter for national and international organizations, along with the development of measurement standards and their intercomparison. As early as 1906, Belot suggested a unit based on the ionizing power of X-rays; in 1908 Villard proposed a unit comprising the liberation of 1 esu of charge per cm³, and in 1912 Christen proposed a unit as energy deposit per unit mass. In 1914, Duane discussed the need for measurements to be made with an 'open-air' (later 'free-air') chamber, and for saturation. In 1918, Krönig and Friedrich provided a comprehensive study of the subject, and other proposals followed.

It was at this juncture that organizations began to play a major role. In the United Kingdom, the Röntgen Society, itself set up in 1897, set up a Committee on Röntgen Measurement and Dosage in 1913, which became the British X-ray Units Committee in 1923 (and continues as BCRU today). It was this latter Committee which was approached by the First International Congress of Radiology (ICR) in 1925 to help set up an International X-ray Units Committee (which continues as ICRU today). By 1928, at the Second ICR the 'Röntgen' was defined in detail as the international unit for the quantity (amount) of X-radiation. Measurement standards to realize this unit were then developed at national standards laboratories, including both 'free-air' and cavity chambers [15.3], and these were subject to international comparison.

In 1937, at the Fifth ICR, the Röntgen was re-defined and included γ-rays as well. At the seventh ICR in 1953, the Röntgen was retained for the measurement of the quantity 'exposure dose', later 'exposure', and a new quantity 'absorbed dose' introduced with its unit the rad. In the 1980s, the introduction of SI units into radiation measurement led to the replacement of the unit rad by the gray, equal to 1 joule/kilogram.

In parallel with the evolution of units of measurement, techniques in clinical dosimetry were developed. Dessauer introduced the use of phantoms in 1912, and with Vierhelle, isodose curves in 1921. Measurements with cavity and condenser chambers became widespread and many individuals made contributions in practical dosimetry.

15.3 Free-air standard chamber in use at the right of the picture developed at the National Physical Laboratory to realise the Röntgen unit (1931).

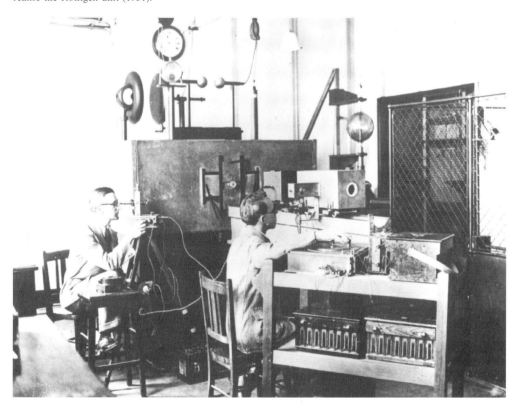

Whether an absolute method is required
Accuracy and precision required
Whether total absorbed dose or absorbed dose rate is required
Whether an immediate read-out is required
Range of absorbed dose to be measured
Range of absorbed dose rate to be measured
Type and energy of radiation to be measured
Need to match dosimeter to medium
Size of detector required
Spatial resolution required
Convenience
Cost
Ruggedness

15.4 Some criteria governing the choice of dosimetric systems (from Boag-Greening, J.R. *Fundamentals of Radiation Dosimetry*, 2nd edn. Adam Hilger, Bristol, 1985).

After the Second World, War, there was a big expansion in all aspects of the subject. Much wider ranges of generating energy, absorbed dose rates and absorbed doses came into use, and these concern protection-level, therapy-level and processing-level requirements. In consequence, existing dosimetric techniques were improved and extended, and many new techniques were developed, such as thermoluminescent dosimetry. The widening range of techniques becoming available led to the opportunity for choice, and [15.4] provides a list of some of the criteria governing such choices.

National Standards Laboratories provided an increasing range of calibration services for exposure (essentially, charge of ions per unit mass of air), absorbed dose (energy imparted per unit mass) and kerma (kinetic energy released per unit mass), along with quantities for use in the measurement of neutrons and radioactivity. Space does not allow for a discussion of the latter quantities. These units are disseminated through networks of Secondary Standard Dosimetry Laboratories, and world-wide uniformity achieved and maintained under the auspices of the International Bureau of Weights and Measures.

Radiological Protection

The ready availability in research laboratories throughout the world of apparatus for studying electrical phenomena in high vacua, and the consequent widespread reproduction during 1896 of Röntgen's discoveries, led also to widespread use of X-rays and, within a short time, widespread appreciation of some harmful effects. Formal action was also speedy and at the meeting of the (British) Röntgen Society on 1 March 1898 a Committee of Inquiry was established to investigate 'the alleged injurious effects of Röntgen rays'. Lead as a protective medium and exposure limitation were already in use by this date, or were being introduced. Lack of a firmly based unit of radiation, however, limited quantitative advice, though in 1902 William Rollins proposed that if seven minutes exposure to X-rays did not fog a photographic plate then the radiation was not of a harmful

intensity. This has been estimated to represent a limit of about 10 röntgens per day.

The rapid spread of diagnostic radiology during the First World War necessitated the widespread dissemination of safety knowledge and the Röntgen Society published recommendations for the greater safety of X-ray operators in 1915. These were followed by similar recommendations from the X-ray Committee of the War Office. Though lacking dose prescription, implementation of the recommendation did require measurement of the absorption coefficients of protective materials and the National Physical Laboratory was asked by the Society to undertake such measurements. The NPL was already involved in X-ray work and had been the recipient in 1913 of the British National Radium Standard, one of a series of international standards constructed to provide a firm base for X-ray dosimetry.

16.1 Harnack-Dean radiographic couch, The Royal London Hospital 1910. Note the absence of protection around the X-ray tubes.

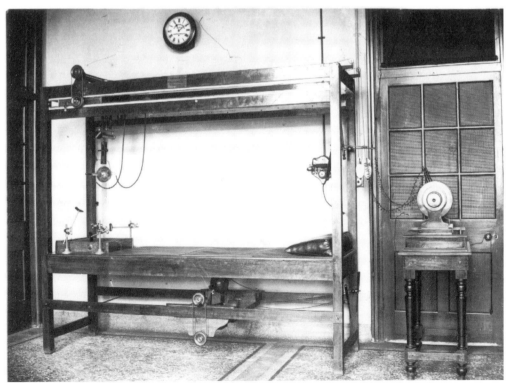

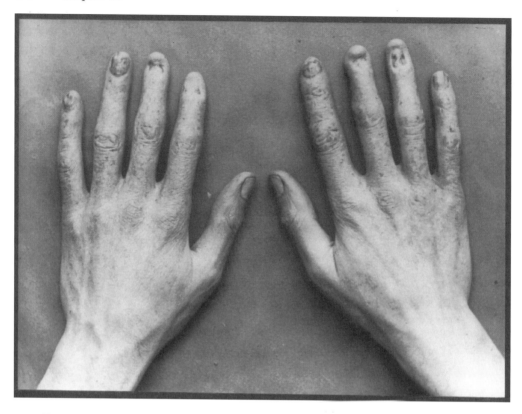

16.2 X-ray dermatitis. The hands of Ernest Wilson, the pioneer radiographer at the Royal London Hospital. Wilson died of his injuries in 1911.

Public concern following press reports of the death of medical personnel from radiation induced cancer resulted, in 1921, in the establishment of a British X-ray and Radium Protection Committee. The Committee issued a preliminary report in July 1921 indicating that the NPL would carry out measurements on protective materials and would also be prepared to inspect facilities; three were inspected that year. The establishment of a tolerance dose for X-radiation was also considered, but due to lack of correlation between physical measurements and biological effects did not form part of the primary protection recommendations. However, inflammation of the skin due to exposure to X-rays was brought within the ambit of factory law in 1924 by its inclusion within the scope of the Workmen's Compensation Act 1906.

London was host to the First International Congress of Radiology at the Central Hall, Westminster, from 30 June to 4 July 1925 when, *inter alia*, it established an International X-ray

Unit Committee. This subsequently changed its name to the International Commission on Radiation Units and Measurements (ICRU). The Physics Section of the Congress placed on record its view as to the desirability of adopting a standard scheme of X-ray and radium protection throughout the world.

At the Second International Congress of Radiology, held in Stockholm in 1928, the views expressed at the First Congress came to fruition when the protective recommendations of the British X-ray and Radium Protection Committee were adopted, with certain minor amendments, as International Recommendations for X-ray and Radium Protection. An

16.3 *right* Newspaper account of the death of Dr Ironside Bruce in 1921 which stimulated the formation of the British X-ray and Radium Protection Committee.

16.4 *far right* Newspaper account of the death of the pioneer radiographer Reginald Blackall in 1925.

Wednesday, March 23, 1921.

DEATH FROM NEW RADIUM TUBES.

NOTED RADIOLOGIST FALLS VICTIM IN PRIME OF LIFE.

DR. IRONSIDE BRUCE.

ANOTHER X-RAY MARTYR IN CAUSE OF HUMANITY.

To the rôle of heroes who have fought and died in the battle of science in the unromantic environment of the science laboratory has now to be added the name of Dr. Ironside Bruce, radiologist to Charing Cross Hospital.

He is yet another of the many martyrs claimed by investigators of the strange, life-giving, yet death-dealing X-rays.

In Dr. Bruce's case death was caused by destruction of the blood, a plastic pernicious anæmia caused by the gamma rays of the new tubes against which the protective measures devised for the older tubes are inadequate.

Pioneer of New Tube.

Dr. Ironside Bruce, who was only 44, was a pioneer in the use of X-ray tubes of higher penetrating power.

An extremely lovable man, he is spoken of in the highest terms by the hospital staff and his

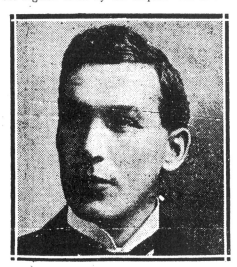

Dr. IRONSIDE BRUCE

assistant, Mr. Curtis, who has worked in close connection with him for 16 years.

Hundreds of letters of sympathy poured in upon his widow to-day from grateful patients all

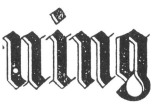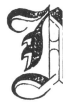

Largest Evening NET S/

N: TUESDAY, DECEMBER 1, 1925.

G THE

MAN WHO GAVE HIS LIFE FOR SCIENCE.

MR. R. BLACKALL'S DEATH AT AGE OF FORTY-FOUR.

15 YEARS X RAY MARTYR.

HANDS AMPUTATED AFTER PIONEER WORK.

The death of Mr. Reginald Blackall, the London Hospital radiographer and X-ray pioneer (reported in last night's *Evening News*) ends a life of wonderful heroism. Mr. Blackall—a martyr to X-rays—died at his home at Leigh-on-Sea. He was only 44 years of age.

Mr. Blackall had suffered from X-ray dermatitis, which results in inflammation destroying the skin, for over 15 years and had undergone no fewer than 20 operations.

He was one of the three pioneers of X-ray work and started at the London Hospital in 1899.

Amputated Hands.

"When Mr. Blackall went to the hospital there was no method of preventing injury to operators, and he undertook the work knowing it would mean death sooner or later," states Mr. Heard, his executor.

"He soon contracted the disease and had to have a finger-nail removed in 1903. Amputation of three fingers followed. He was so ill in 1920 that he had to retire from active work, but at his own request still acted in an advisory capacity.

"The disease had spread so much three years later that both Mr. Blackall's hands had to be amputated, but he never complained, and set to work to learn to write with an artificial hand so that he

MAI

A HAI

Mr. J
Nelson,
experin
whethe
during

He is
to New
summer

If it is
into be
exceptic
ments
Austral
exchan;

EIGI

DAILY

Eight
ing var
Free I
Daily I
The :
paid by

which
paid fo
Detai
been a
Mail I
Domini
below.

KI

£250 N

International (X-ray and Radium) Protection Committee, later to be renamed the International Commission on Radiological Protection, was also established to be responsible for exchanging views and presenting suggestions for revision of the recommendations to the next Congress. The problem of international inter-comparison of doses was resolved when the Congress adopted an International X-ray Unit of Intensity.

Further modifications to the International X-ray and Radium Protection Committee's recommendations were agreed at the Third International Congress in Paris in 1931, and at the Fourth in Zurich in 1934 when a tolerance dose of 0.2 international röntgens per day was set. At Chicago in 1937 the Fifth Congress extended the application of the tolerance dose to the gamma rays from radium, and restated the limit as 0.2 R/day or 1 R/week. Systematic measurement of occupational doses by films or condenser chambers was recommended and, as a result, the NPL introduced film monitoring using dental films for its staff.

World-scale international collaboration came to an end during the Second World War. However, as in the First World War, concern at the increasing uses of ionizing radiations resulted in a more widespread dissemination of protective recommendations. Whereas in the past such recommendations had been in the form of advice, concern over hazards in luminizing with radium-based paint led to the introduction of mandatory provisions through the factories (Luminizing) (Health and Safety Provision) Order, 1942. In the same year, the Ministry of Health asked the NPL to extend film monitoring to hospitals, and the following year HM Chief Inspector of Factories requested a further extension to industry, including luminizers. Other monitoring laboratories were in operation, but such monitoring did not have to be continuous. Under the Factories (Luminizing) Special Regulations, 1947, for example, the occupier was required to make arrangements for the wearing of a suitable photographic film in one week in every period of three months, and was required to maintain records indicating whether or not such films appeared to have been exposed to radiations exceeding one röntgen in the aggregate. Medical examinations at regular intervals (three monthly from 1942, monthly from 1947) were the main personal control.

Although the dangers of ingestion, inhalation, skin contamination and external radiation had been present in the luminizing industry, and from earlier days during the separation of radium from its ore, work on the production of the atomic bomb and the development of artificial radionuclides intensified some aspects

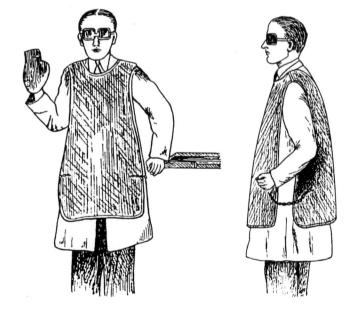

16.5 Observers protective smock (A.E. Barclay, *The Digestive Tract* 1933). Barclay comments that this smock was better than the old design of apron which was supported by a strap around the neck and which the operator took off as soon as the authorities back was turned!

of these dangers, so the provision of 'health physics' advice and services became a major focus of attention during the Manhattan Project. Proposals for the relative biological effectiveness of other radiations relative to that of X-radiation and for maximum permissible body burdens and airborne concentrations for particular nuclides were formulated, and at a Tripartite Conference at Chalk River in 1949 the scope of maximum permissible dose limitation was extended to include special provision for the hands and forearms. These concepts were included in revised recommendations from the International Commission on Radiological Protection which was reformed and renamed at the Sixth International Congress of Radiology, held in 1950 for a second time in London. In these recommendations the maximum permissible whole body was reduced from 1 R per week to 0.5 R per week al the surface of the body, which was taken as corresponding to 0.3 R per week in free air.

As a result of a reorganization in Great Britain, the British X-ray and Radium Committee handed over its responsibilities to the Medical Research Council and the Minister of Health. In 1953 the Radiological Protection Service (RPS) was formed and subsequently took over the personnel monitoring and some other services from NPL. A further revision of ICRP recommendations took place in 1954, and in 1957 general guidance based on these recommendations was issued to hospitals in the Health Service in the form of a Code of Practice for the Protection of Persons exposed to Ionizing Radiations. A revision of this Code, renamed 'Code of Practice for the Protection of Persons against Ionizing Radiations arising from Medical and Dental Use' followed further revised ICRP recommendations in 1958 (ICRP Publication 1); a sister code for Research and Teaching was also introduced. In addition all industrial users were brought under legislative control by the Ionizing Radiations (Sealed Sources) Regulations 1961. These documents incorporated the revised ICRP occupational dose limit of $5(N-18)$ rem where N is the age in years, with the additional stipulation that the dose accumulated during any 13 consecutive weeks should not exceed 3 rem.

Following the next ICRP revision (ICRP Publication 9), which dropped the age-related dose formula as the main limit in favour of a straight 5 rem in a year maximum permissible dose, industrial provisions were further refined by the Ionizing Radiations (Unsealed Radioactive Substances) Regulations 1968 and the Ionizing Radiations (Sealed Sources) Regulations 1969. A further reorganization of advisory and service provision in 1970 saw the RPS amalgamate with the Radiological Protection Division of the United Kingdom Atomic Energy Authority's Health and Safety Branch to form the National Radiological Protection Board (NRPB).

When the ICRP next revised its recommendations in 1977 (ICRP Publications 26) and explicitly developed a system of dose limitation

---

Role of NRPB

Central to the medical uses of radiation are the judgements, skills and concern of doctors, scientists and radiographers, supported by other health professionals. NRPB's role is summarized here.

NRPB
Collaboration with professionals in radiology
Interaction with international organizations
Formal advice on patient protection
National medical radiation surveys
Scientific papers, meetings and exhibitions
Information to the media and public
Technical services
    Radiation protection advisor
    Personal monitoring
    Dental monitoring
    Training

16.6 The role of the NRPB (National Radiological Protection Board).

involving justification and optimization in addition to dose limits, the UK was a member of the European Community, and it was necessary for revised legislation to comply with the EC legislation which followed this publication (EC Council Directive 80/806/Euratom). The Health and Safety at Work etc. Act 1974 extending legislation to all workers was also in force, and this provision was included in the subsequent legislation, the Ionizing Radiations Regulations 1985. An Approved Code of Practice accompanied the regulations and additional information on good radiation protection practice consistent with regulatory requirements was included in 'Guidance notes for the protection of persons against ionizing radiations arising from medical and dental use', which followed much of the format of the previous codes of practice. A further EC Council Directive laying down basic measures for the radiation protection of persons undergoing medical examination or treatment (84/46/Euratom) has been implemented by the Ionizing Radiation (Protection of Persons Undergoing Medical Examination or Treatment) Regulations 1988.

The latest revision of ICRP's recommendations (ICRP Publication 60, 1991), which recommend an occupational dose limit of 20 mSv per year averaged over defined periods of 5 years, has still to be introduced into legislation. NRPB, in accordance with a direction by the Health Ministers to advise the appropriate government departments and statutory bodies on the acceptability of such recommendations to, and on their application in, the United Kingdom, has published a Board Statement (Doc NRPB, 4, No 1). Further guidance in relation to occupational, public and medical exposures has been given (Doc NRPB, 1, No 2). Representatives from the UK are engaged in discussion with representatives from the other Member States on the revision of Directive 80/806/Euratom.

A report on patient dose reduction in diagnostic radiology was issued by the Royal College of Radiologists and the NRPB in 1990 (Doc NRPB, 1, No 3). Other NRPB documents have been issued concerning clinical magnetic resonance diagnostic procedures, protection of the patient in X-ray computed tomography, and on diagnostic medical exposures to ionizing radiation during pregnancy. These complement initiatives within the European Community to develop reference doses and quality criteria in diagnostic radiology.

100 Years of Radiobiology

Biological effects were noted very soon after Röntgen discovered X-rays in Germany in 1895. The following year in the USA Dr Daniels noted hair loss in a colleague following irradiation and this led to the successful treatment of a benign hairy naevus in 1897 by Leopold Freund in Vienna. Experimental radiobiology soon followed and in 1903 Heinecke observed the interphase death of lymphocytes. In 1906 Bergonié and Tribondeau noted that cells in the rat testis were more 'radiosensitive' if they were mitotically active. Nowadays the term radioresponsiveness would be applied to their data. The quantitative measure of *radiosensitivity* had to await the clonal survival assay of single mammalian cells developed by Puck and Marcus in 1955.

Meanwhile, radiotherapists like Coutard had shown in 1919 that the surrounding normal tissues could tolerate more radiation if the dose to the tumour was fractionated. Reisner used skin erythema measurements in 1932 to confirm that skin recovered from radiation damage during fractionated radiotherapy. In 1944 Magnus Strandqvist had used such fractionation data to show that, for given levels of skin

damage, isoeffect curves would fit a straight line on a log-log graph of increasing dose and overall time [17.1]. Frank Ellis developed this concept in 1965 to give separate weight to the number of fractions of a course of radiotherapy, as well as its overall time. As an alternative, Douglas and Fowler showed in 1976 that the dose response of skin to different numbers of fractions of radiation can be explained by a linear-quadratic model.

From the start radiobiologists used model systems. Hermann Muller found a dose-response for mutation rates using the Drosophila fruit fly in 1927. Experimental mice were also used extensively. In 1935 Mottram showed that cells in tar warts were more damaged by radiation if they were nearer the vascular supply. That observation suggested a correlation of radiation response with the oxygen tension of the tissue and this was confirmed by Hal Gray, Oliver Scott and their team in 1953. Tikvah Alper and Paul Howard-Flanders used bacteria to show their *K* curve of increasing cellular radiosensitivity with oxygen concentration in 1956.

Cellular radiobiology was revolutionized in 1956 when Puck and Marcus used their single cell survival technique to show that the radiation

17.1 Iso-effect curves relating the total dose and overall treatment time for skin tolerance (from Strandqvist, 1944)

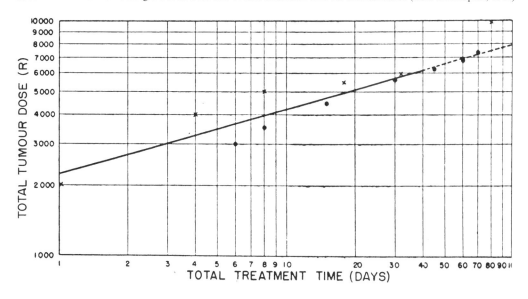

dose-response curve of mammalian cells is exponential apart from an initial shoulder [17.2]. The shape of the survival curve provided a measure of the radiosensitivity of different cells irradiated under different conditions. The shoulder on the curve was explained by Mortimer Elkind and Harriet Sutton in 1959 in terms of repairable sub-lethal radiation damage. In 1961 the cell survival technique was used by Toyozo Terasima and Leonard Tolmach to show that radiosensitivity varied at different times during the division cycle. That cycle had been delineated by Alma Howard and Stephen Pelc in 1953 when they showed that there is a discrete central phase of DNA synthesis; this is the S phase.

Nuclear bombs were dropped over Hiroshima and Nagasaki in 1945 and by 1952 Folley and colleagues showed an increased incidence of leukaemia in the survivors. This confirmed that radiation can be carcinogenic but Arthur Upton showed in 1961 that the dose-response curve is bell-shaped [17.3]; i.e. low doses are relatively more carcinogenic because cells do not survive higher doses. In 1957 William Court Brown and Richard Doll had found a high incidence of leukaemia in patients irradiated with low doses for ankylosing spondylitis. In 1954 Liane and William Russell had shown that embryopathy is another hazard and described how the pattern changes with time during pregnancy when mouse embryos are irradiated.

At a fundamental level, Douglas Lea made a mathematical analysis in 1946 of cell survival in terms of the inactivation of targets by radiation. Pulse radiolysis was used by John Boag and Edward Hart to demonstrate the hydrated electron in 1963. In the same year Gerald Adams and David Dewey showed that chemicals with an affinity for electrons would act as radiosensitizers, in the same way as oxygen. In 1976 Dieter Frankenburg identified DNA double strand breaks as the lethal lesion in a repair deficient yeast. In 1988 John Savage showed that sister-chromatid exchanges can only be detected in human lymphocytes after densely ionizing radiation. As early as 1940, L.H. Gray had shown that such radiation has a relatively higher biological effectiveness and is much less influenced by oxygen than X-rays.

The exponential shape of the radiation dose response curve was found to apply to every type

17.2 Radiation dose-response of human cancer cells in terms of survival of colony-forming ability in vitro (from Puck and Marcus, 1956)

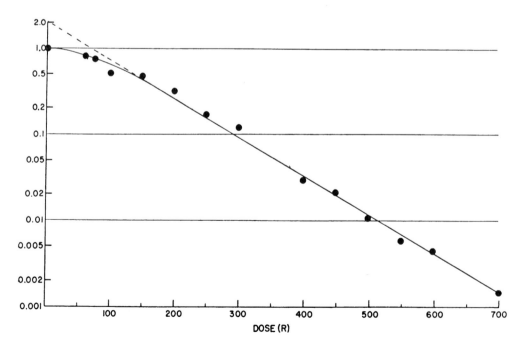

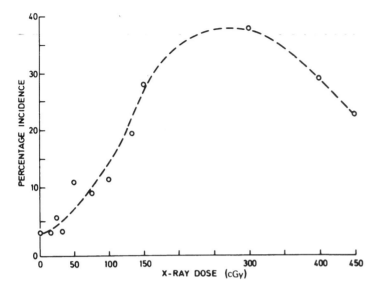

17.3 Dose response for the incidence of myeloid leukaemia in mice following total body irradiation (from Upton 1961)

of mammalian tissue for which a cellular assay could be devised. Many of these used experimental mice. Harold Hewitt and Charles Wilson showed this for leukaemic cells in 1959. James Till and Edward McCulloch used a spleen colony assay for normal bone marrow cells in 1961. Rodney Withers found it for regenerating skin stem cells in 1967 and, with Mortimer Elkind, for intestinal stem cells in 1970. In 1986 Jolyon Hendry and Howard Thames developed the concept of tissue-rescuing units and pointed out that the radiation dose-response of these tissues can be related to their content of such units.

Experimental radiotherapists applied all this radiobiology to the design of the optimal treatment of human tumours. In 1981 Bernard Fertil and Edmond Malaise showed that the radiation

response of such tumours can be correlated with the shape of their cell survival curve over the low dose range. In 1982 Rodney Withers demonstrated a systematic difference in the effect of fractionating the dose to tissues depending on whether they show an early or a late response to radiation. He also raised the question in 1988 whether the rate of tumour cell proliferation may accelerate after radiotherapy, as had been shown for normal skin by Juliana Denekamp in 1973. When Trott and colleagues analyzed the dose-effect curves from skin cancer patients in 1984 they confirmed that the therapeutic ratio between tumour control and skin necrosis is much reduced for larger tumours [17.4].

Towards the end of this century of radiobiology there have been contributions from

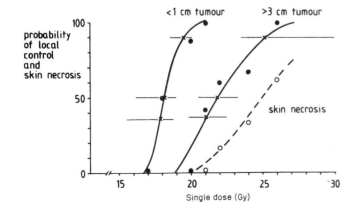

17.4 Dose effect curves for the control of skin cancers of different size compared with skin necrosis (from Trott *et al* 1984)

molecular genetics. Malcolm Taylor showed in 1975 that patients with ataxia telangiectasia can be extremely radiosensitive because of the failure of their cells to repair radiation damage. Finally, Larry Thompson cloned the first gene for radiosensitivity to be found in human cells— XRCCl.

Dental Radiology

'To what perfection, gentlemen, may not the science and art of dentistry reach if some of the new things which press upon your attention are fully realized. Already painless dentistry is within your grasp by aid of electricity and simple anaesthetics, and now the X-ray more than rivals your exploring mirror, your probe, your most delicate sense of touch, and your keenest powers of hypothetical diagnosis'

William J. Morton, 24 April 1896
Address to the New York Odontological Society

The practice of dentistry is largely, if not exclusively, concerned with the prevention, diagnosis and treatment of diseases affecting the teeth and jaws. Therefore it is no surprise to find that the potential of Professor Röntgen's discovery of X-rays in dentistry was quickly recognized. Morton's words readily demonstrate the enthusiasm felt by many dentists about the new 'X-ray light'. It is uncertain who took the first dental radiograph, but the honours are most fairly shared between the Germans Koenig and Walkhoff, the eminent Sheffield dentist Frank Harrison and C. Edmund Kells of New Orleans, all of whom were producing crude but recognizable dental 'skiagrams' in the late winter and early spring of 1896.

Initially there was no such thing as a 'Dental X-ray set'; equipment was either homemade or adapted from medical use. Harrison described dental radiography as a 'scientific obstacle race' using gas tubes and induction coils, while many pioneer dental radiographers report the unpredictability of the X-ray output from such equipment. The first commercial 'dental' X-ray set was not marketed until 1905, by the predecessors of Siemens in Germany. Radiation doses were initially very high: Harrison, in an address to the Midland Counties branch of the British Dental Association in June 1896, reported using exposure times ranging from 6 to 40 minutes for intra-oral films. This was fairly typical, and Harrison was probably the first to report a radiation injury from dental radiography. An assistant, exposed to a number of X-ray examinations over a four week period, suffered subsequent progressive facial pain, erythema, desquamation and hair loss.

In 1898 William Rollins, a dentist from Boston, Massachusetts, carried out some animal experiments which demonstrated that 'X-light' could cause burns or even death. Nevertheless some pioneer dental radiologists, notably Kells, maintained the safety of X-rays well into the 1900s. Indeed, some claimed a therapeutic value for radiation in cases of 'pyorrhoea'. Ironically Kells was ultimately to fall victim to severe radiation induced injuries and cancer, contributing to his death in 1928. Operator and assistant injuries to hands were not uncommon in dental radiography, not only because of the practice of 'setting the tube' by using their own hands, but also due to holding films and plates for the patient. The belief of the German dentist Schaeffer-Stuckert (1897), that '...neither with an apparatus nor by the patient himself can the film be pressed so closely to the palate as by the fingers of a second person', was widely held.

Early dental radiographers took both extraoral and intraoral radiographs. However, as Schaeffer-Stuckert's words imply, radiography in the mouth presented pioneer dental radiologists with some unique problems: difficult access, an awkwardly shaped cavity, copious amounts of moisture and control of head and tongue movement. Although conventional glass plates were used outside the mouth, they were less successful for intraoral use because of the problems of cutting very small plates without damaging the emulsion, their fragility and patient discomfort. Both Harrison in Sheffield and Morton in the United States experimented successfully with Eastman Kodak roll film. In the early 1900s the Seed Dry Plate Company produced a celluloid base dental film supplied in large sheets; these were cut to size by the user and sealed in gutta-percha or wrapped in rubber for protection against moisture. This method of protecting films from moisture and light continued to be used until 1919, when the first commercially produced machine-wrapped dental film, Kodak Regular, was introduced.

Exposure times for dental radiographs were reduced to about 8 seconds using this film.

Despite the widespread practice of the operator holding the film, other dentists designed film holders to aid stability and support the film. These ranged in complexity from mounting the film in impression compound (Harrison's 'contrapshun' of 1896), through a clever design modified from a dental mirror [18.1], to complex designs incorporating devices to correctly angle the X-ray beam. The development of the bisecting-angle technique by the Pole Cieszynski in 1907, whereby a satisfactory shadow of a tooth can be cast onto the film by using careful beam angulation, did much to rationalize the previously erratic technique of intra-oral radiography; it remains widely used today.

The introduction of the Coolidge tube, in the second decade of this century, permitted the production of more predictable X-ray exposures and a higher output. It is interesting to note that Coolidge owed something of his design to a dentist, the American William Rollins. Coolidge referred extensively to the latter's *Notes on X-ray Light* published in 1904. A second major improvement in dental X-ray set design was the introduction of the first 'shockproof' machine (the Victor CDX) by General Electric in 1923. Prior to this design, high voltage wires were exposed (as was the X-ray tube) and the risk of electric shocks to both patients and operators high. The 'shockproof' design placed all the high tension wires and tube in an oil-filled chamber, acting to improve both electrical and radiation safety. Nevertheless, open-tube designs [18.2] continued to be produced into the 1930s.

In 1896, Harrison stated pessimistically that 'this work is altogether too complicated and to expensive to be added to the dental outfit'. Sure enough, until the commercial production of dental X-ray equipment and machine-wrapped film dental radiography remained the pursuit of an enthusiastic minority of dentists. However, the 1920s and 1930s saw a steady rise in the numbers of dentists using X-rays as a diagnostic aid. At the same time improvements in film speed and equipment design led to improved quality with lower radiation doses. In 1924, the double-sided emulsion for dental film was introduced, immediately halving radiation doses, while speed was further reduced by Kodak in 1940, 1955 and 1980. Non-screen film remains the most widely used image receptor in dental radiography today, with the fastest currently available film (E-speed) permitting exposure times of less than half a second to be readily achievable. Increasingly, the paralleling technique for periapical radiology using special film holders and a longer focus/film

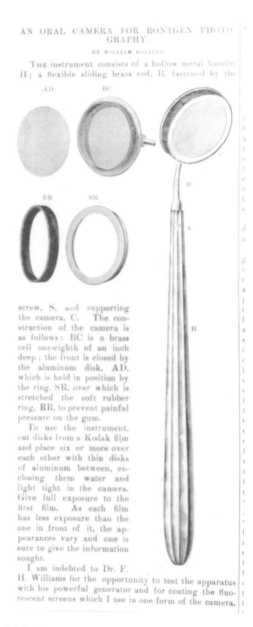

AN ORAL CAMERA FOR RONTGEN PHOTOGRAPHY.

BY WILLIAM ROLLINS.

THE instrument consists of a hollow metal handle, H; a flexible sliding brass rod, B, fastened by the screw, S, and supporting the camera, C. The construction of the camera is as follows: BC is a brass cell one-eighth of an inch deep; the front is closed by the aluminum disk, AD, which is held in position by the ring, SR, over which is stretched the soft rubber ring, RR, to prevent painful pressure on the gum.

To use the instrument, cut disks from a Kodak film and place six or more over each other with thin disks of aluminum between, enclosing them water and light tight in the camera. Give full exposure to the first film. As each film has less exposure than the one in front of it, the appearances vary and one is sure to give the information sought.

I am indebted to Dr. F. H. Williams for the opportunity to test the apparatus with his powerful generator and for coating the fluorescent screens which I use in one form of the camera.

18.1 The Rollins intraoral cassette (1896), based on a dental mirror. A round piece of film was fitted into the cassette which formed the head of the instrument.

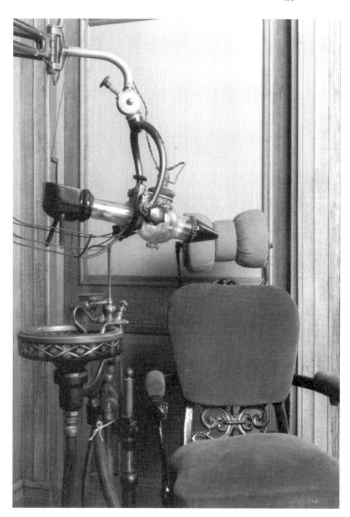

18.2 A Ritter X-ray unit (1928), incorporating a Coolidge tube with exposed high-tension wires.

distance, propounded by McCormack in 1937, is replacing the bisecting angle technique leading to improved image quality. At the same time, the introduction of higher kilovoltage X-ray sets with improved collimation has led to considerable reductions in patient dose.

Dentists often desire a 'full mouth' radiographic survey of patients, achieved traditionally by taking multiple intraoral radiographs. The theory of panoramic radiography of the jaws was independently developed by Numata in Japan in the 1930s and Paatero in Finland in the 1940s. Essentially a modified form of tomography, an image of both jaws can be produced on a single film. Panoramic equipment is now produced by many manufacturers and is widely used by general dental practitioners.

In the face of rapid advances in medical imaging, dental radiography is often perceived as a technological backwater, using simple low-powered X-ray equipment and nonscreen film. In the last five years this impression has been changed by the introduction of digital intraoral X-ray systems using charge-coupled devices such as the receptor [18.3]. Other systems using photostimulable plates are currently being developed for dental use. Many new panoramic X-ray machines incorporate complex software to allow the production of precise cross-sectional images of the jaws for use in implantology. The establishment of a Diploma in Dental Radiology by the Royal College of Radiologists in the 1980s and the recognition of the subject as a dental specialty have done much

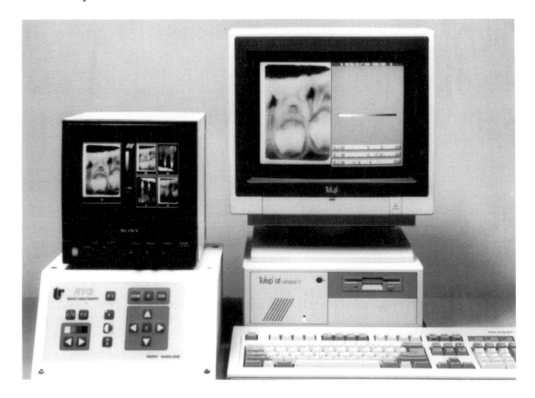

18.3 A modern digital intraoral radiography system using a charge-coupled device as image receptor.

to raise standards of dental radiological teaching and clinical services.

Today, radiography carried out by dentists makes up about a quarter of all medical radiological examinations in the United Kingdom, with around 15 million made annually in England and Wales alone. While research has demonstrated that the reliability of radiology in diagnosis of dental diseases is not the 'gold standard' that Morton anticipated in 1896, it remains an essential tool of all dentists. After one hundred years, the dental profession continues to have cause for considerable gratitude for Röntgen's discovery of 'A New Kind of Rays'.

19

Radiology in Scotland

Scots have claimed credit for many important inventions and discoveries in the last two centuries but not, of course of X-rays. However, it was the reputation of a Scots scientist, Lord Kelvin, that led Röntgen to send him a copy of his classic paper on the properties of X-rays. Kelvin gave the paper to his brother-in-law, J.T. Bottomley, an associate of Lord Blythswood and John Macintyre [19.1] in electrical experiments.

Macintyre, whose mother, Margaret Livingstone, was a relative of the explorer David, was a specialist in ear, nose and throat medicine in Glasgow Royal Infirmary. His fame, however, rests on his interest in electrical engineering. With J.T. Bottomley and Lord Blythswood, he gave the first of three demonstrations on X-rays to the Philosophical Society of Glasgow on 5 February 1896, only three weeks after A.A.C. Swinton's claim to have produced the first

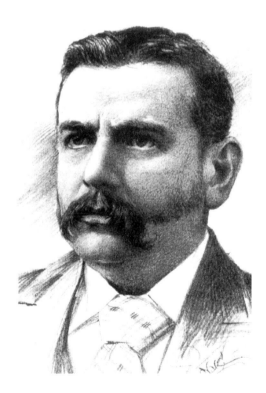

19.1 Dr John Macintyre 1857–1928

radiograph of a human hand in Britain. Macintyre's electrical department [19.2], opened in Glasgow Royal Infirmary in February 1896, was the first radiological department in the county and possibly in the world. Macintyre's work included the first radiographs of soft tissues of thorax [19.3] and abdomen, of a kidney stone, of a coin in the oesophagus and of a bullet in the human body. One of his most famous innovations was, in 1897, his ciné radiograph of a moving frog's leg, the first time bones moving within a living creature had been studied.

Early in his career, Macintyre observed that skin reactions from early X-rays were common. This caused him to insist on stringent protective measures, making him a pioneer of radiation safety. This observation also prompted him to begin treating tumours with X-rays.

Silvanus Thomson, the first President of the Röntgen Society, referred in his presidential address in 1897 to the early pioneers in radiology by saying, 'to particularise might be invidious but none will object to my mention of Dr Macintyre of Glasgow.........who was one of the earliest and most successful practitioners of the new art.'

Doctors in other centres in Scotland were also early to take an interest in X-rays. On the same day that Bottomley, Blythswood and Macintyre gave their paper in Glasgow, Dawson Turner demonstrated photographs taken by the Rontgen process to a meeting of the Edinburgh Medico-Chirurgical Society. His photograph of a purse with two metallic clips, containing a florin and a key, shown at this meeting is now among a collection of Dawson Turner's X-rays in the Museum of the Royal College of Surgeons, Edinburgh.

In November 1896, Dawson Turner was appointed Assistant Medical Electrician to the Royal Infirmary, becoming Electrician in 1901. He suffered severe radiation burns which eventually caused the loss of three fingers and an eye. He died on Christmas Day 1928 and his name is recorded on the Martyrs' Memorial at St George's Hospital, Hamburg.

In Aberdeen, James McKenzie Davidson, originally an ophthalmologist, is another with

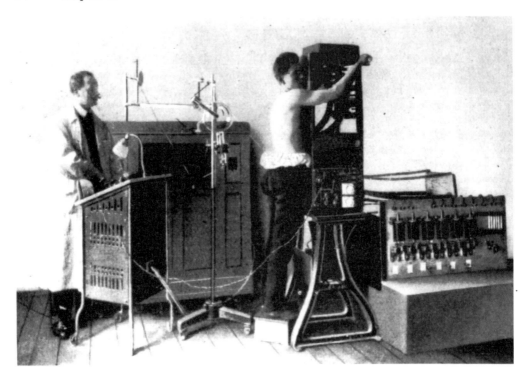

19.2 Dr Macintyre's Electrical Pavilion. Glasgow Royal Infirmary, *c.* 1897.

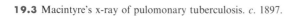
19.3 Macintyre's x-ray of pulomonary tuberculosis. *c.* 1897.

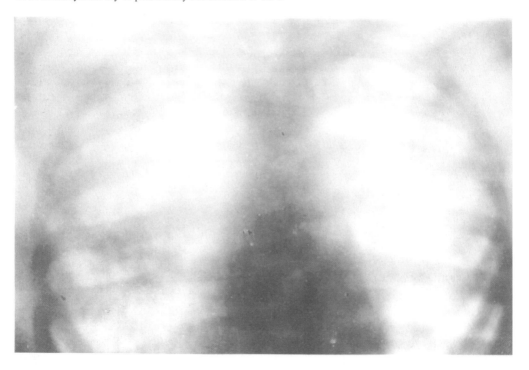

good claim to have produced the first radiographs in Scotland. He is famous for having produced a device for the X-ray localization of intra-ocular foreign bodies. He went to London in 1897 to become Britain's leading radiologist of the day and was subsequently knighted. His work in Aberdeen was taken on by John Levack who was appointed Medical Electrician in 1896 and, in 1919, Lecturer in Radiology and Therapeutics.

In Dundee, George Pirie was appointed in 1896 to superintend the Electrical Medicine Department, where he developed both diagnostic and therapeutic radiology. He died, in 1929, an early martyr to radiology.

The work of the early pioneers was carried on by many others too numerous to list but mention of a few names helps to illustrate developments.

In Glasgow's Western Infirmary, Donald J. Mackintosh was a contemporary of the other early workers and became Medical Electrician in 1896. He was particularly interested in fractures and dislocations and published his *Atlas of Skiagraphy*' in 1899. In 1920, he was succeeded by James R. Riddell. During his time, contrast media examinations were introduced and X-ray films replaced photographic plates. Riddell died of radiation burns and sarcoma, like Turner and Pirie, a martyr to radiology and one of the first 16 names on the Martyrs' Memorial [19.4]. He was succeeded by J. Struthers Fulton and by S.D. Scott Park in 1940. This was the beginning of the modern era which saw separation of diagnostic radiology from radiotherapy in 1946, the establishment of an angiographic service in 1954 and Ian Donald's pioneering work in ultrasound in the late 1950s. It is interesting that the author, along with many of his fellow students, was unimpressed by Donald's early ultrasound pictures. Little did he know that

19.4 The names of Drs Pirie and Riddell on the Martyrs' Memorial, Hamburg.

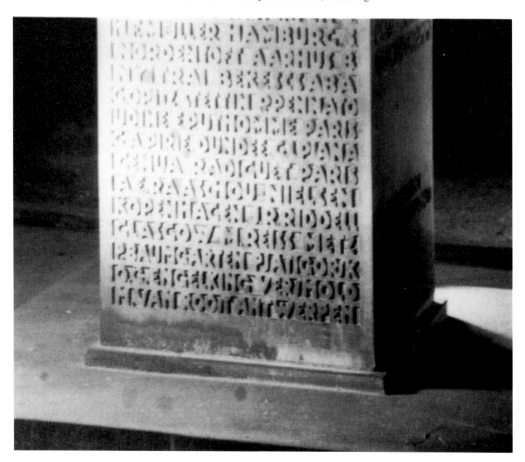

ultrasound would subsequently play such a large part in his working life.

In Aberdeen, John Blewett, appointed first whole time Head of Department and Henry Griffith, first Honorary Physicist, developed the photographic monitoring of radiation exposure, now familiar to all who work in places where radiation is a hazard.

The Department of Medical Physics in Aberdeen, under Professor John Mallard, developed the world's first whole body MRI scanner in 1980 (at the same time the University of Nottingham developed a head scanner).

The early workers were both diagnostic radiologists and radiotherapists. (Sir) George Beatson, a pioneer of cancer treatment was a surgeon who became famous for demonstrating the effectiveness of oophorectomy in breast cancer. He became first Director of the Glasgow Cancer Hospital in 1894. This hospital subsequently moved to larger premises in 1896 and expanded further in 1912 when it became the Glasgow Royal Cancer Hospital. In 1928, Dr Peacock, Director of the Research Laboratory at the hospital was given £10 000 by Lady Burrell for the purchase of half a gram of radium.

Following visits to the Middlesex Hospital and the Curie Foundation in Paris, Peacock established the Radium Institute. It agreed to lend radium to other institutions provided they agreed to a uniform plan of treatment, record keeping and statistical publication.

In 1952, the Glasgow Royal Cancer Hospital was renamed the Royal Beatson Memorial Hospital. In 1966 it was amalgamated with the units at the Western and Royal Infirmaries to become the Glasgow Institute of Therapeutics. Today, the Beatson Oncology Centre, now based at the Western Infirmary, is the second largest cancer treatment centre in the United Kingdom.

Radiologists from both disciplines in Scotland are still united by membership of the Scottish Radiological Society. The Society developed

19.5 *Left to right*
Professor Robert Steiner, Warden of the Faculty of Radiologists
Professor Edward McGirr, President, RCPSG
Professor (later Sir) Howard Middlemiss, President of the Faculty of Radiologists
Dr Hunter Cummack, President of the Scottish Radiological Society
at a joint meeting in Glasgow in 1972.

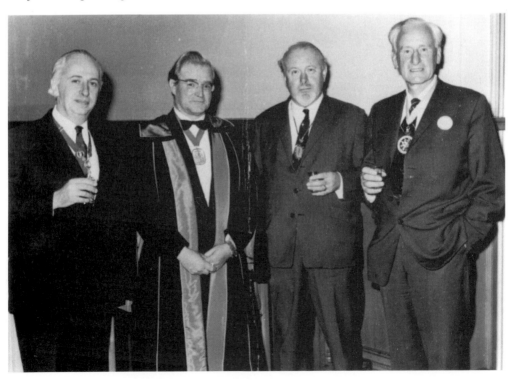

from being a Scottish section of the British Institute of Radiology to being constituted a separate society on 21 September 1946, with 15 members present. The first Chairman was Dr David Levack of Aberdeen. In 1947 it was agreed that an annual subscription of five shillings would meet all expenses.

Since its inception, the Society has held scientific meetings in different venues throughout Scotland [19.5]. It also awards prizes and scholarships and has an annual lecture in memory of Dr John McGibbon, a pioneering cardiac radiologist from Edinburgh.

After almost half a century, the Society with a membership of over 300, anticipates continuing its special role in furthering radiology in Scotland.

Radiology in Ireland: The Early Years

When the news of the amazing new scientific discovery reached Ireland in early January 1896, some dozen laboratories had the requisite apparatus to generate X-rays. That Professor John Joly FRS [20.1], of Trinity College Dublin, could give formal advance notice that he would demonstrate the 'new Lenard or Röntgen Rays' at a meeting of the Dublin University Experimental Association on 15 February 1896 implied that he was experimenting with the subject since sometime in January. At that lecture he demonstrated a number of photographs he had taken with Lenard rays, including one showing the bones of his own hand.

Belfast was equally quick off the mark: on 24 February 1896, Dr Cecil Shaw gave a lecture on the new Röntgen Rays to the Ulster Amateur Photographic Society; he showed a number of X-ray photographs, including one demonstrating disease in the bones of a hand due to 'blood poisoning'.

On 16 March 1896 at the request of Surgeon Bolton McCausland, a fragment of needle in a girl's hand was demonstrated radiographically by Professor Barrett and Mr Jefcote at the Royal College of Science Dublin. The fragment was successfully removed and McCausland's report in the *British Medical Journal* 28 March 1896 was the first clinical report of the application of the new rays from Ireland. On 13 April 1896 a broken needle in a woman's hand was demonstrated by Brother Potamian O'Reilly at the De La Salle College in Waterford and, on 28 May, a bullet lodged in a man's thigh was localized on X-rays taken at Queen's College, Cork. Many laboratories, hospitals, professional photographers and chemists were producing X-rays on a regular basis for clinical purposes before the end of 1896.

The man most responsible for demonstrating the clinical potential of X-rays and establishing radiology as a recognized clinical discipline was William Steele Haughton [20.2], though he remained a practising surgeon all his career. He was truly the Thurstan Holland of Irish radiology, whom he anticipated in radiological practice by some two months. Before the end of

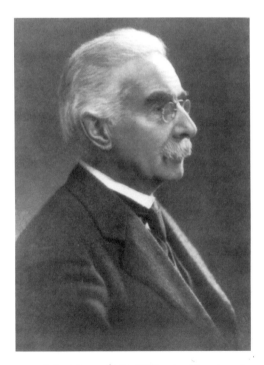

20.1 John Joly FRS (1857–1933), scientific polymath; co-founder Irish Radium Institute.

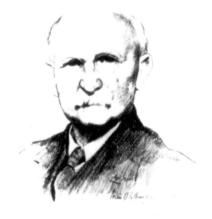

20.2 W.S. Haughton (1869–1951), Dublin X-ray pioneer.

March 1896, he was using his own X-ray apparatus, first at Sir Patrick Duns Hospital and, after 1900, at Dr Steeven's. His first paper to the Royal Academy of Medicine in Ireland on 7 May 1897 was based on 150 cases during the previous 14 months and was a clear comprehensive review of the clinical applications of X-rays at that time. The range of material was quite remarkable: it included tuberculosis of bones and joints, fractures, foreign bodies in the trachea and oesophagus, and a series of radiographs illustrating epiphyseal development at the hand, wrist and elbow from 3 to 18 years; the reproductions in the journal are clear and sharp indicating the high quality of the original radiographs. He also demonstrated movements of the cervical spine, heart and diaphragm on a fluorescent screen and warned that prolonged or repeated short exposures could cause dermatitis.

During the next 6 years, Haughton lectured to many learned societies on X-rays and, by March 1902, he had X-rayed over 1 900 patients; he could discuss the application of fluoroscopy in phthisis, acute pneumonia, emphysema, pleurisy, pneumothorax, aneurysms and intrathoracic tumours and was using bismuth subnitrate in the oesophagus and stomach. Haughton was generous in imparting his expertise to others, including Surgeon-Major John Battersby. Battersby's experience in examining casualties after the Battle of Omdurman in July 1898 established the position of X-rays in military surgery.

By November 1896, the Royal Hospital in Belfast had acquired its own X-ray apparatus and contracted with a local firm of chemists to provide a clinical service at the hospital. This arrangement, first with Clarkes and then with Lizars, lasted until 1903. Initially, some of the Dublin hospitals used a professional photographer but, by 1898, virtually all the Dublin hospitals had their own apparatus. The Queen's Colleges at Cork and Galway X-rayed patients for local doctors from mid-1896, and so did some secondary colleges such as Clongowes Wood.

John Rankin's [20.3] career in Belfast paralleled that of Haughton in Dublin: his interest in X-rays dated from his student days in 1899 and he was appointed 'Medical Electrician' to the Royal Victoria Hospital in 1903. For two decades, he provided, single handedly, a growing combined diagnostic and therapeutic service,

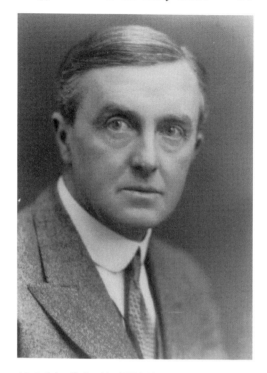

20.3 John C. Rankin (1876–1954), Belfast X-ray and radiotherapy pioneer.

though he never relinquished his other interests in venereology and bacteriology. His paper in the *Archives of the Röntgen Rays* in 1906 on 'The treatment of malignant diseases by X-rays' was an important paper on the subject and his *Atlas of Skiagrams Illustrating the Development of Teeth* (with Symington) was an important milestone in radiological anatomy.

Rankin was joined in 1920 by Maitland Beath who developed an international reputation and was President of the British Association of Radiologists in 1938/39, when he played an important role in the transformation to the Faculty of Radiologists. Frank Montgomery returned to Belfast in 1924 and built up the radiotherapy services; his services to medicine in Northern Ireland were recognized by a knighthood in 1953.

During the first decade of Irish radiology, all of the exponents devoted only part of their time to X-rays but, by 1900, formal hospital appointments were being made, usually termed 'medical electricians'—E.J.M. Watson to Sir Patrick Duns in 1900, C.M. Benson to Baggot Street in 1902, J.C. Rankin to the Royal Victoria

Belfast in 1903, W.C. Stevenson to Dr Steevens in 1904, James Meenan to St Vincent's in 1905. The next decade was marked by the advent of fulltime career radiologists,—Maurice Hayes at the Mater from 1907, Garrett Hardman at the Richmond from 1912 and Michael O'Hea at Vincent's from 1913. The 1920s saw the return of formally qualified radiologists with the Cambridge Diploma, such as Frank Montgomery to Belfast in 1924 and John Geraghty to Dublin in 1926.

Many early radiologists were also interested in the therapeutic uses of X-rays and of radium, notably Walter Clegg Stevenson, whose collaboration with John Joly resulted in the formation of the Irish Radium Institute in 1914. Joly had conceived the idea of enclosing the radium 'emanations' (radon) in fine glass capillaries, which was done by R.J. Moss, a chemist and skilled glass-blower. The capillaries, inserted within exploring needles, provided a more uniform radiation of tumours and thus was born the Dublin Method of Radium Therapy.

The early radiographers were largely self-taught but, as the discipline developed, it became evident that specific training was necessary. Ralph Leman in Belfast started training radiographers in 1926 and a formal training program was established there in 1930. A School of Radiography was set up in St Vincent's Hospital Dublin in 1931. All the programmes, at Dublin, Belfast and later Derry, complied with the requirements of the College of Radiographers and have in recent years progressed to degree courses in radiography. A training programme for radiologists

was set up in Belfast in the mid-1950s and, since then, over 120 radiologists have been trained in the scheme, the majority emigrating when qualified.

In 1932, the Radiological Society of Ireland was formed and it was entirely appropriate that Haughton should be unanimously invited to become its first President, which he remained until his death in 1951. Another milestone in the development of Irish radiology was the establishment of the Faculty of Radiologists of the RCSI in 1961 and, from the start, there was close and cordial collaboration between the new Faculty and the London Faculty (and later the RCR), including reciprocity of Part I examinations for the respective Fellowships.

The Faculty has been involved in undergraduate and postgraduate instruction in radiology and its success in promoting academic radiology is illustrated by the presence of five chairs of radiology in Irish medical schools. In 1967, the Irish Faculty set up its own postgraduate training programme for radiologists; until then Ireland was dependent on Britain for training its radiologists, especially during the post-War decades when there was a dramatic expansion of radiological services throughout Ireland. The Faculty has also been active in radiological education in the Middle East.

The association between Irish and British Radiology has always been close and cordial, with frequent combined meetings of Irish and British societies. The generous assistance from many British radiologists and departments has been very much to the benefit of radiology in Ireland.

Radiological Organizations in the United Kingdom

The British Institute of Radiology [21.1]

Following initial private meetings on 18 March, 1897 and later on 2 April 1897, it was agreed that a society for the study of the newly discovered X-rays was needed. An advertisement was placed in the *British Medical Journal* for 10 April announcing the formation of the

society with David Walsh as the Honorary Secretary. From the first it was decided that the society was not just for medical people and 'should include all who are interested in the scientific study of the Röntgen Rays.' The first general meeting was on 3 June and the formal inaugural meeting of the Röntgen Society was held on 5 November at St Martin's Town Hall with Silvanus Thompson as President and

21.1 The development of the British Institute of Radiology and the College and Society of Radiographers.

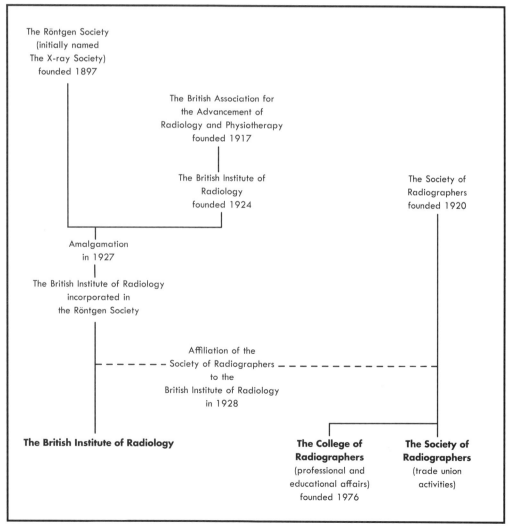

Professor W.C. Röntgen and Sir William Crookes as Honorary Members.

By 1917 the need for a university examination in radiology for doctors became apparent. The British Association for the Advancement of Radiology and Physiotherapy was founded and the Diploma in Medical Radiology and Electrology (DMRE) at the University of Cambridge was set up. This diploma could be taken by external students. This purely medical body was not strong financially and was assisted by the Röntgen Society. This body became the British Institute of Radiology in 1924 and amalgamated with the Röntgen Society in 1917. The need for a separate medical organization was still felt and ultimately resulted in the formation of the Faculty of Radiology.

The British Institute of Radiology was responsible for the first International Congress of Radiology held in London in 1925 with Thurstan Holland as President. The BIR also encouraged the formational of the Society of Radiographers and inspired the work of the X-ray and Radium Protection Committee.

In 1927 the Röntgen Society and the British Institute of Radiology were amalgamated to form the modern British Institute of Radiology. The BIR was incorporated by Royal Charter in 1958 and Royal Patronage was bestowed in 1979.

The Section of Radiology, the Royal Society of Medicine [21.2]

The Royal Society of Medicine was founded in 1907 by the amalgamation of a number of medical societies. One of these specialist societies was The British Electro-Therapeutic Society which had been founded in 1902 and continued from 1907 as the Electro-Therapeutic Section. The Electro-Therapeutic Society was a purely medical organization in distinction to the Röntgen Society. The Royal Society of Medicine moved to its current location at 1 Wimpole Street in 1912. In 1931 the Electro-Therapeutic Section became the Section of Radiology. A Section of Oncology was formed in 1970.

The Royal College of Radiologists [21.3]

In the 1930s the need for medical radiological organizations was apparent and the British

21.2 Radiology in the Royal Society of Medicine.

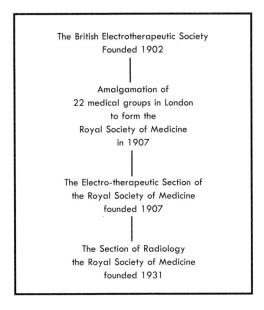

The British Electrotherapeutic Society
Founded 1902

Amalgamation of
22 medical groups in London
to form the
Royal Society of Medicine
in 1907

The Electro-therapeutic Section of
the Royal Society of Medicine
founded 1907

The Section of Radiology
the Royal Society of Medicine
founded 1931

Association of Radiologists (1934) and the Society of Radiotherapists of Great Britain and Ireland (1935) were formed. They joined forming the Faculty of Radiologists in 1939. At that time it was felt inappropriate for a further college to be formed. The new Faculty was supported by the Royal Colleges. A charter was granted in 1953. A supplementary charter was granted in 1975 and the Royal College of Radiologists was created. In 1990 two College faculties of Clinical Radiology and Clinical Oncology were formed.

The Institute of Physical Sciences in Medicine [21.4]

The Hospital Physicists' Association (HPA) was founded in 1943 following a meeting at the British Institute of Radiology. Prior to the formation of the HPA the salary of the hospital physicist was settled by local personal negotiation. The Association established itself nationally and internationally through its journal, its meetings and its publications. In 1977 the Hospital Physicists' Association was registered as an independent trade union and in 1982 the Institute of Physical Sciences in Medicine (IPSM) was formed. This change in name reflects the fact that not all members are associated with

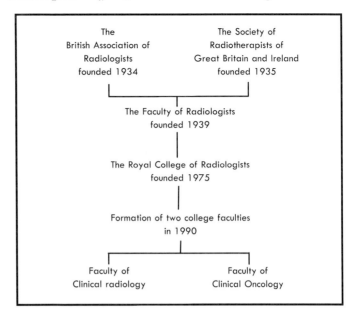

21.3 The Royal College of
Radiologists

hospitals. The IPSM consists of the Institute of
Physical Sciences in Medicine dealing with scientific
activities and publications and the Hospital
Physicists' Association looking after professional
and trade union activities. In 1993 the Hospital
Physicists' Association merged with the Manu-
facturing, Science and Finance (MSF) Union.

The Scottish Radiological Society

Before the Second World War there were

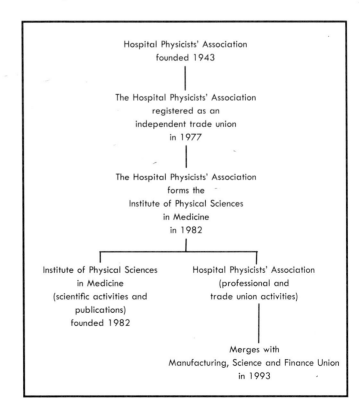

21.4 The Institute of Physical
Sciences in Medicine.

meetings of the Scottish Section of the British Institute of Radiology. In 1946 there was consultation amongst radiologists in Scotland as to the form of meetings and as a result the Scottish Radiological Society was formed, without affiliation to any other society. The society had a scientific and social role, as well as the power to deal with matters political and administrative. From 1954 the executive council which dealt with the political aspects of the Society was made responsible to the Society with equal representation of therapy and diagnosis. In 1970 the Society acquired a permanent address at the Royal College of Physicians in Queen Street Edinburgh. The Society's representative role was taken over by the Scottish Standing Committee of the Faculty of Radiologists, now the Royal College, following health service reorganization in the 1970s. Scientific meetings of the Society have continued with many joint meetings with scientific bodies in the UK and abroad.

The Society and College of Radiographers

In 1920, under the Presidency of Sir Archibald Reid, The Society of Radiographers was incorporated with the objects of promoting and developing the science and practice of radiography, and study and research in it; also to protect the honour and interests of radiographers. First examinations were held in 1921 and the first successful candidates from the examination were admitted to membership in March 1921. By 1935 sufficient progress had been made to enable the Society to publish a monthly professional journal *Radiography*, now known as *Radiography Today*. The first Fellowship examinations were held in 1937.

After the inception of the National Health Service the Society was invited to be part of the Staff Side negotiating committee, the Whitley Council thereby helping to develop its negotiating role for radiographers. In 1960 the Professions Supplementary to Medicine Act was passed and with it state registration for radiographers through the Radiographers Board.

Because of potential problems arising from the Society's charitable status and its industrial relations role, the Society formed The College of Radiographers in 1976 as a wholly owned private company registered as a charity and taking as its objects the professional and educational objects of the Society, leaving it the responsibility for industrial relations for the combined organization. The Society affiliated to the TUC in 1991.

Graduate education for radiographers was started in the UK in 1989 and by 1993 the profession was wholly graduate entry.

The Society and college celebrate their 75th Anniversary in 1995. Membership has grown from 30 in 1920 to 13 500 in 1994.

Selected Bibliography

Andrew ER. Magnetic resonance imaging: a historical overview. In: *Encyclopedia of Nuclear Magnetic Imaging*. New York: Wiley in press.

Blume SS. *Insights and Industry*. Cambridge, Massachusetts: The MIT Press, 1992.

Brewer AJ. *Classic Descriptions in Diagnostic Roentgenology*. Springfield: Charles Thomas, 1964.

Bull JWD. History of neuroradiology. *British Journal of Radiology* 1961, **34**: 69–84.

Burrows EH. *Pioneers and Early Years: A History of British Radiology*. Alterney: Colophon Press, 1986.

Bushong SC. *The Development of Radiation Protection in Diagnostic Radiology*. Boca Raton, Florida: CRC Press, 1973.

Caufield C. *Multiple Exposures: Chronicles of the Radiation Age*. London: Secker & Warburg, 1989.

Eisenberg RL. *Radiology, An Illustrated History*. St Louis: Mosby Year Book, 1992.

Geddes LA & Geddes LaNE. *The Catheter Introducers*, Chicago: Mobium Press, 1993.

Goldberg BB & Kimmelman BA. *Medical Diagnostic Ultrasound: A Retrospective on its 40th Anniversary*. Rochester, USA: Kodak Health Services, 1988.

Grigg ERN. *The Trail of the Invisible Light: from X-Strahlen to Radio(bio)logy*. Springfield: Charles Thomas, 1965.

Jordan MA. *The Maturing Years*. London: The College of Radiographers, 1995.

Levak I & Dudley H. *Aberdeen Royal Infirmary: The People's Hospital of the North East*. London: Balliere Tindall, 1992.

Mayneord WV. Some applications of nuclear physics to medicine. *British Journal of Radiology* 1950, Supplement No 2.

Moodie I. *50 Years of History*. London: The Society of Radiographers, undated.

Mould RF. *A Century of X-rays and Radiography in Medicine*. Bristol: Institute of Physics Publishing, 1993.

Mourino MR. From Thales to Lauterber, or from the lodestone to MR imaging: magnetism and medicine. *Radiology* 1991; **180**: 593–612.

Pallardy G, Pallardy M-J & Wackenheim A. *Histoire Illustrée de Radiologie*. Paris: Les Éditions Roger Dacosta, 1989.

Quimby EH. The history of dosimetry in röntgen therapy. *American Journal of Roentgenology*, 1945; **54**: 688–703.

Rowbottom M & Susskind C. *Electricity and Medicine: History of Their Interaction*. London: Macmillan Press, 1984.

Viega-Pires JA & Grainger RG. *Pioneers in Angiography: the Portuguese School of Angiography*, 2nd edn. Lancaster: M.T.P. Press, 1987.

Webb S. *From the Watching of Shadows: the Origins of Radiological Tomography*. Bristol: Adam Hilger, 1990.

The British Journal of Radiology 1993; **46**: No 550. Special Issue to Celebrate the 75th Anniversary of the British Institute of Radiology.

Seminars in Nuclear Medicine 1970; **IX**: No 3. Special Issue on Selected Historical Aspects of Nuclear Medicine.

History of the Hospital Physicist's Association 1943–1983. Newcastle-upon Tyne: The Hospital Physicist's Association, 1983.

Contributors

W.F. BLAND is at the National Radiological Protection Board

J.F. CALDER is a Consultant Radiologist at the Victoria Infirmary, Glasgow, UK

J.E. DACIE is a Consultant Radiologist in the Department of Diagnostic Imaging, St Bartholomew's Hospital, London, UK

R. DICK is Head of Radiology, Royal Free Hospital, London, UK

J.E.E. FLEMING is in the Department of Obstetrics and Gynaecology, University of Glasgow, Glasgow, UK

R.G. GRAINGER is Kodak Professor Emeritus of Diagnostic Radiology, University of Sheffield, UK

J.M. GUY is a Consultant Radiologist at the Yeovil District Hospital, Yeovil, Somerset, UK

K. HALNAN was formerly Director of Radiotherapy and Oncology, Royal Postgraduate Medical School, Hammersmith Hospital, London, UK

K. HORNER is Head of the Unit of Oral and Maxillofacial Radiology, University of Manchester, Manchester, UK

R.K. INGRAM is Head of the School of Radiography, Oxford Centre for Radiographic Studies, Cranfield University, UK

J.D. IRVING is Honary Senior Lecturer in Radiology, Royal Postgraduate Medical School, University of London, UK

I. ISHERWOOD is Professor Emeritus of Diagnostic Radiology, University of Manchester, Manchester, UK

M. JORDAN is former Chief Executive of the College of Radiographers

W.A. JENNINGS was formerly Head of the Division of Radiation Science and Acoustics, National Physical Laboratory, Teddington, Middlesex, UK

R.F. MOULD, Scientific Consultant, Surrey, UK

J.P. MURRAY is Professor Emeritus of Diagnostic Radiology, University College, Galway, Ireland

A.H.W. NIAS is Emeritus Richard Dimbleby Professor of Cancer Research, University of London, London, UK

E.B. ROLFE is a Consultant Neurologist at the Queen Elizabeth Hospital, Edgbaston, Birmingham, UK

E.M. SWEET was formerly Consultant Radiologist at the Royal Hospital for Sick Children and the Queen Mother's Hospital, Glasgow, UK

A.M.K. THOMAS is a Consultant Radiologist in the Department of Diagnostic Imaging, Bromley Hospital, Bromley, UK

N. TROTT Emeritus Reader in Physics as applied to Medicine, Institute of Cancer Research, University of London, UK

S. WEBB is in the Joint Department of Physics, Institute of Cancer Research and Royal Marsden Hospital, Sutton, Surrey, UK

P.N.T. WELLS is Honorary Professor of Clinical Radiology, University of Bristol, Bristol, UK

B. WORTHINGTON is Professor of Diagnostic Radiology, University of Nottingham, Nottingham, UK.

Index